CRAZY AMBULANCE STORIES

VOLUME 2

DEREK CHANCE

FREE REIGN
Publishing

ISBN 13: 979-8-89234-110-3

Free Reign Publishing, LLC
San Diego, CA

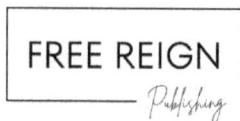

FREE REIGN
Publishing

CONTENTS

INTRODUCTION

Welcome to the wild and unpredictable world of emergency medical services as seen through the eyes of veteran paramedic Derek Chance. In *Crazy Ambulance Stories*, Derek takes you on a thrilling ride through the most bizarre, heart-pounding, and sometimes downright hilarious incidents he's encountered during his 15 years on the job. From high-speed chases to unexpected rescues, each story offers a unique glimpse into the life of a paramedic, where every call could be the difference between life and death, and no two shifts are ever the same. With his signature blend of humor, compassion, and raw honesty, Derek invites you to buckle up and experience the adrenaline-fueled adventures that make up his daily reality. Get ready for a series that will make you laugh, cry, and appreciate the unsung heroes of emergency medical services.

CHAPTER ONE

CHILD LEFT IN A HOT CAR

THE DISPATCH CAME in at 14:27 on what had to be the hottest day of the year. The sun was a merciless beast, beating down on the city with an intensity that turned concrete into a frying pan and air into a sauna. We were just returning from a relatively routine call when the alert blared through the radio, sending us hurtling toward the scene.

"Child left in a hot car," the dispatcher announced. My heart sank, and I felt that familiar cocktail of adrenaline and dread. I pushed the ambulance faster, the siren blaring as we wove through traffic. These calls never got easier, no matter how many times I'd responded to them.

We arrived at a supermarket parking lot, where a small crowd had gathered around a sweltering sedan. The windows were fogged with condensation, an ominous sign. I grabbed the necessary equipment and hustled over to the car. Bystanders had managed to get the door open, and I reached in to lift the child out. The heat inside the vehicle was like opening an oven door, the oppressive wave slapping me in the face.

The patient was limp, skin flushed and hot to the touch. My training kicked in immediately. This was heat-stroke, a dire emergency. I quickly assessed the situation: rapid, shallow breathing, a weak but palpable pulse, and a glassy-eyed, semi-conscious gaze. I motioned for my partner to bring over the stretcher and started our rapid sequence of treatment.

We whisked the patient into the cool confines of the ambulance, the blessed air conditioning offering a brief respite from the relentless heat. I initiated cooling measures right away, stripping down the patient's clothing to allow maximum skin exposure. Cool, damp towels were placed on the head, neck, and groin—major blood vessels areas—to speed up the cooling process.

I grabbed an IV setup and inserted the needle with practiced precision. Normal saline began to flow, helping to rehydrate and stabilize blood pressure. Heatstroke can cause severe dehydration, which leads to a drop in blood pressure and a risk of organ failure. The saline would help counteract this, buying us precious time.

Next, I affixed the cardiac monitor leads to the

patient's chest. The heart rate was elevated, as expected, but there were no arrhythmias. This was a small relief. Heatstroke often leads to heart complications, but so far, the patient's heart was holding steady under the strain.

I then placed a pulse oximeter on the patient's finger. Oxygen saturation was a bit low, likely due to the hyperventilation, so I adjusted the oxygen mask to deliver a steady flow of supplemental oxygen. This would help ensure that the brain and vital organs received the oxygen they desperately needed.

My partner and I worked in a seamless dance of efficiency, each move practiced and precise. The patient needed more than just cooling and hydration; we had to monitor for seizures and other complications. Heatstroke can cause the brain to swell, leading to seizures, and in severe cases, brain damage. I prepared a dose of midazolam, a benzodiazepine, ready to administer if any seizure activity started.

While monitoring the patient's condition, I kept my movements steady and calm, despite the rising tension. The situation was dire, but panic had no place in the back of an ambulance. Every second counted, and my focus was razor-sharp. The patient's body temperature had to be brought down quickly to prevent further damage.

We kept the ambulance cool, the air conditioning on

full blast. I continued to switch out the damp towels, replacing them with fresh, cold ones as they warmed against the patient's skin. The patient's breathing started to slow, becoming more regular, a sign that our efforts were beginning to take effect.

As we barreled down the road toward the hospital, I glanced at the vital signs monitor. Heart rate was still high, but stable; blood pressure was holding, and the patient's oxygen levels were improving. We were making progress, but I knew better than to relax. Heatstroke is a treacherous enemy, and complacency can be deadly.

I checked the IV site for any signs of infiltration or blockage, ensuring that the fluids were flowing freely. The saline solution was vital, not just for rehydration, but for helping to cool the patient from the inside out. I could see the beads of sweat forming on the patient's skin, a good sign that the body was starting to regulate its temperature again.

Time seemed to stretch and compress in the back of the ambulance. We were moving at high speed, but every second felt like an eternity. I kept my focus on the patient, monitoring every slight change in condition, ready to respond at a moment's notice.

We finally arrived at the hospital, and I gave a rapid report to the awaiting emergency department staff. The patient was still unconscious but showing signs of improvement. We transferred the patient onto a hospital stretcher, and the medical team quickly took over, continuing the cooling and monitoring processes we had started.

As I stepped back, the gravity of the situation hit me again. The heatstroke could have easily been fatal, but we had managed to stabilize the patient, giving them a fighting chance. I took a deep breath, the tension slowly releasing from my body as I handed over the last bits of information to the ER team.

Back in the ambulance, my partner and I shared a look. No words were necessary; we both knew the importance of every moment in cases like this. I started the paperwork, detailing the events and treatment provided. It was a necessary part of the job, but my mind was still partially with the patient, hoping for a positive outcome.

Despite the severity of the call, I couldn't help but find a moment of dark humor as I scribbled down my notes. This job, with its high stakes and emotional rollercoasters, often required finding the lighter side, even if it was just for a fleeting second. Maybe it was a defense mechanism, a way to cope with the harsh realities we faced daily.

I finished the report and closed the file. Another call would come soon enough, another crisis to manage, another life to save. For now, I allowed myself a moment to breathe, to appreciate the small victories amidst the chaos.

We drove back to the station, the sun still blazing outside but feeling just a little less oppressive now. The patient's chances were good, thanks to quick action and effective treatment. As a paramedic, that's all I could hope for—to make a difference, one call at a time.

CHAPTER TWO

A TRUE BLACK EYE

IT WAS JUST another evening shift when the call came in, an urgent dispatch about a man who had attempted to inject black dye into his eye. I read the details twice, just to be sure. The things people do never cease to amaze me. My partner and I jumped into the ambulance and sped toward the address.

When we arrived, we found the patient in his small, cluttered apartment. He was sitting on the floor, clutching his face with one hand, the other holding a syringe. The syringe was empty, but the evidence of his attempt was painfully clear. Black fluid oozed from the corner of his eye, staining his cheek and dripping onto his shirt. I took a deep breath and reminded myself to remain professional.

I approached the patient carefully, assessing his condition. His eye was already beginning to swell, and the area around it was an angry shade of red. His pupil was dilated, and the sclera was stained with streaks of black. He was in obvious pain, wincing and moaning softly. I could see that the situation was serious, but I couldn't help but think about how absurd it was. Who in their right mind tries to inject dye into their eye?

The first step was to stabilize the patient and get him to the hospital as quickly as possible. I asked him to lie down on the stretcher. He complied, though it was clear every movement caused him discomfort. I quickly hooked him up to the necessary monitors. His vital signs were stable, but his heart rate was elevated, likely due to the pain and panic.

I cleaned the area around his eye as best as I could with saline solution. It wasn't much, but it was crucial to remove as much of the dye as possible. The patient flinched at the touch of the cold saline, but it was necessary. I noted the color and consistency of the dye. It was an oily, viscous substance, clearly not meant for injection, let alone into an eye. The risk of infection was high, and I knew we had to act fast.

As I continued to clean the eye, I checked for any signs of a foreign body. Thankfully, the syringe seemed to have been the only object involved. I irrigated the eye thoroughly, using copious amounts of saline. The dye was stubborn, but I managed to clear most of it. The patient's eye was still a mess, but at least it wasn't as black as it had been.

Next, I applied a sterile dressing to the eye to protect it during transport. The patient's discomfort was palpable, but he remained surprisingly cooperative. I started an IV line to administer pain relief and antibiotics. The latter was crucial to prevent the almost certain infection that would follow such an ill-advised act. I could see the relief wash over him as the pain meds began to take effect.

We secured the patient on the stretcher and loaded him into the ambulance. As we sped towards the hospital, I continued to monitor his vital signs. His heart rate had come down slightly, but his blood pressure was still elevated. I kept a close eye on his oxygen saturation, though it remained stable. The real concern was the potential damage to his eye and the risk of systemic infection from the dye.

I used the time to document everything. The patient's initial presentation, the treatment provided, and his response to it. It was essential to have a detailed record for the doctors at the hospital. I also noted his apparent mental state. While he was clearly distressed, there was no sign of disorientation or confusion. He was aware of what he had done, and though he hadn't explained why, it was clear he regretted it.

Halfway to the hospital, the patient began to

mumble. The pain relief had taken effect, and he seemed more relaxed. His eye was still a mess, but the swelling had stabilized. I continued to irrigate the eye periodically with saline, trying to keep it as clean as possible. Every so often, I would catch a glimpse of the black dye still present in the sclera, like an inkblot on paper.

The patient's other eye remained unaffected, which was a small blessing. I could only imagine the horror if he had attempted to inject both eyes. I tried to keep things light-hearted, despite the seriousness of the situation. After all, humor is a good coping mechanism. I thought about how this incident would make for an interesting story in the break room, though I'd leave out any identifying details.

The hospital came into view, and I radioed ahead to let them know what we were bringing in. An ophthalmologist would need to be on standby, and they'd need to prepare for possible surgery. The patient's eye was at serious risk, and they'd need to act quickly to save as much of his vision as possible.

As we pulled into the emergency bay, I felt a sense of relief. The patient was stable, and we'd done everything we could to mitigate the damage. I knew the doctors would take it from here. We carefully transferred the patient from the ambulance to a gurney, ensuring his eye was still protected. The ER team took over, asking for a quick summary of what had happened.

I provided the details, emphasizing the urgency of the situation. The ophthalmologist was already on his way, and the ER team moved swiftly. I watched as they wheeled the patient away, feeling a mix of satisfaction and curiosity. I'd likely never know why the patient had done what he did, but I hoped he'd get the care he needed and learn from this painful experience.

Back in the ambulance, I cleaned up and restocked, ready for the next call. I couldn't help but chuckle at the absurdity of the situation. It was just another day on the job, dealing with the unexpected and the inexplicable. As we headed back out, I couldn't shake the image of that inky black eye, a bizarre reminder of the lengths people go to for reasons known only to them.

CHAPTER THREE

TAKING A BATH

I WAS NEARING the end of my shift when the call came in: a morbidly obese woman was stuck in her bathtub and couldn't get out. Calls like this were not uncommon, but they always presented unique challenges. I grabbed my gear and headed to the ambulance, my partner already behind the wheel, ready to go.

Upon arrival at the scene, we were greeted by the patient's frantic family. They had tried everything to help her out but had no success. The patient's home was a modest, single-story house with narrow hallways and small rooms—certainly not designed for easy maneuvering of a stretcher or medical equipment. We made our way to the bathroom, which was located at the end of a tight hallway.

The patient was in her late 50s, weighing approximately 450 pounds, and had been stuck in the bathtub for several hours. She was visibly distressed and in pain. Her skin was pale and clammy, and she was breathing heavily, signs that she was in significant distress. We immediately took stock of the situation. The bathroom was small, with barely enough space for us to maneuver. The patient was wedged in the tub, her legs swollen and discolored from prolonged immobility and poor circulation.

We began by assessing her vital signs. Her blood pressure was elevated, likely due to the stress and discomfort, reading at 180/110 mmHg. Her heart rate was tachycardic at 110 beats per minute, and her oxygen saturation was slightly below normal at 92%. Given her obesity, we were concerned about the possibility of respiratory distress and other complications.

To complicate matters, the patient had a history of type 2 diabetes, hypertension, and chronic lymphedema. Her legs were massively swollen, and there were signs of cellulitis, a bacterial skin infection, which required immediate attention. We knew we had to act quickly and efficiently to prevent further complications.

First, we administered supplemental oxygen via a nasal cannula to help improve her oxygen saturation. We then focused on her pain management. Given her size and the difficulty in accessing a vein, we opted for intramuscular injection of pain relief medication. We chose ketorolac, a non-steroidal anti-inflammatory drug, which would help reduce her pain and inflammation.

Next, we needed to extricate her from the bathtub. This was no small feat. We called for additional support from the fire department, as we would need more manpower and possibly specialized equipment to lift her safely. In the meantime, we used blankets and towels to provide some cushioning and to help us get a better grip. The fire department arrived with an air cushion device, designed to help lift heavy patients. We carefully positioned the cushions around the patient and slowly inflated them, creating enough space for us to slide her onto a backboard.

With great effort and coordination, we managed to lift the patient from the tub and onto a stretcher. This required precise timing and communication to ensure her safety and prevent further injury. Once she was securely on the stretcher, we began moving her out of the bathroom. Navigating the narrow hallway was tricky, but with the help of the fire department, we managed to get her into the living room where there was more space to work.

During the transport to the ambulance, we continued to monitor her vital signs and provided reassurance to keep her calm. Her oxygen levels improved slightly, but her heart rate remained elevated. We maintained her on supplemental oxygen and kept a close eye on her condition.

Once we got her into the ambulance, we performed a more thorough assessment. We noted signs of potential deep vein thrombosis (DVT) in her legs due to the prolonged immobility and poor circulation. This was a serious concern, as a clot could dislodge and travel to her lungs, causing a pulmonary embolism. We decided to administer low-molecular-weight heparin, an anticoagulant, to reduce the risk of clot formation. We also started an intravenous line to ensure we had access for fluids and medications if needed during the transport.

The ride to the hospital was relatively smooth. We continued to monitor her condition closely. Her pain was somewhat managed, but she remained uncomfortable due to her size and the constraints of the stretcher. We did our best to keep her stable and reassured, knowing that her anxiety could exacerbate her symptoms.

Upon arrival at the hospital, we provided the emergency department staff with a detailed handover, including her medical history, the circumstances of the incident, and the treatments administered. They quickly took over, preparing to address her immediate medical needs, including the cellulitis, potential DVT, and her overall physical condition.

As we left the hospital, I reflected on the challenges we faced during this call. The patient's obesity added layers of complexity to an already difficult situation, requiring us to use all our skills and resources to ensure her safe extrication and transport. Despite the difficulties, we managed to get her to the hospital without any major complications, which was a testament to the teamwork and dedication of everyone involved.

In conclusion, dealing with a morbidly obese patient stuck in a bathtub required not just physical effort but also careful medical assessment and intervention. From managing her pain and breathing to addressing the risk of blood clots and infections, every step needed to be carefully planned and executed. It was a challenging call, but one that underscored the importance of preparedness and teamwork in emergency medical services.

CHAPTER FOUR
HEAD ON COLLISION

THE CALL CAME in just after 2 AM, the radio crackling with the urgency of the dispatcher's voice. "Head-on collision with a telephone pole, vehicle versus fixed object. Possible severe injuries. Respond immediately." My partner, Jackson, and I exchanged a quick glance, both of us feeling the adrenaline surge. We had been through countless emergencies together, but every call carried its own unique blend of dread and anticipation.

We sped through the deserted streets, the siren's wail slicing through the night. As we approached the scene, the flashing lights of police cruisers and fire trucks illuminated the wreckage. The car, a compact sedan, was crumpled around the telephone pole like a discarded soda can. Steam hissed from the ruptured radiator, and the acrid smell of gasoline and burnt rubber filled the air.

We grabbed our gear and made our way to the vehicle. The driver's side was a twisted mess of metal and glass, but the patient was still conscious, pinned behind the steering wheel. The windshield was a spiderweb of cracks, and blood trickled from a gash on the patient's forehead. The front airbags had deployed, their deflated forms hanging limply.

My initial survey began with a quick assessment of the scene for any immediate dangers. The pole had held firm, but the car was precariously balanced. Jackson was already communicating with the fire department to stabilize the vehicle while I focused on the patient.

The patient's face was pale, lips tinged blue, indicating potential hypoxia. I noted the absence of a seatbelt, which likely exacerbated the injuries. Breathing was rapid and shallow, with the chest rising unevenly. A quick check of the pulse revealed it was weak and thready, a sign of possible shock.

I slipped on my gloves and reached for the trauma shears, carefully cutting away the clothing to expose the injuries. There was an obvious deformity in the right leg, likely a femur fracture, and the left arm was bent at an unnatural angle. A deep laceration on the forehead was the source of the bleeding, but what concerned me more was the possibility of a traumatic brain injury given the mechanism of the collision.

While Jackson worked with the firefighters to extricate the patient, I applied a cervical collar to immobilize the spine. We couldn't rule out a spinal injury given the high-impact nature of the crash. Next, I placed an oxygen mask over the patient's face to assist with breathing, adjusting the flow to 15 liters per minute.

Once the firefighters had pried the door open with the Jaws of Life, we carefully lifted the patient onto a backboard, securing them with straps to prevent any further movement. The extrication was delicate and time-consuming, but we finally had the patient free and ready for transport.

Inside the ambulance, I continued my assessment. The patient's Glasgow Coma Scale (GCS) score was concerningly low at 8, indicating a severe head injury. Pupils were unequal, another red flag for intracranial pressure. I quickly started two large-bore IV lines, one in each arm, and began administering fluids to combat the shock.

A rapid secondary survey revealed additional injuries. The abdomen was distended and tender, suggesting internal bleeding. I applied a pelvic binder to stabilize any potential pelvic fractures. The left arm had an open fracture, bone fragments protruding through the skin, necessitating immediate care to prevent infection and further blood loss.

I monitored the patient's vital signs closely, noting any changes. Blood pressure was dangerously low, heart rate erratic. I relayed all findings to the hospital via radio, alerting them to prepare for a trauma code on arrival. My hands moved almost on autopilot, performing tasks that had become second nature after years of experience.

The ride to the hospital felt both interminably long and blindingly fast. Every bump and turn was a potential threat to the patient's precarious condition. I administered pain relief and anti-nausea medication, careful to monitor the patient's responses. Jackson kept the vehicle steady, his focus unwavering despite the chaos around us.

As we neared the hospital, the patient's condition took a turn for the worse. Blood pressure continued to drop, and the pulse became more irregular. I prepared for potential cardiac arrest, setting up the defibrillator and ensuring we had all necessary medications at hand.

We arrived at the emergency department in a whirlwind of motion. The trauma team was ready and waiting, and we quickly transferred the patient to their care. I provided a rapid handover, detailing the injuries and treatments administered. The doctors and nurses moved with practiced efficiency, their focus now on saving the patient's life.

As I stepped back, the adrenaline began to fade, replaced by the familiar exhaustion of a high-stakes call. Jackson and I exchanged a look of grim satisfaction, knowing we had done everything in our power to give the patient the best possible chance.

I cleaned and restocked the ambulance, preparing for the next call. There was always another emergency waiting, another life hanging in the balance. The job was relentless, but moments like these reminded me why I had chosen this path. Every life saved, every crisis averted, was a testament to the skill and dedication of the team. And for now, that was enough.

In the aftermath of the call, the details of the patient's injuries replayed in my mind. The head-on collision with the telephone pole had caused significant trauma, and the initial survey had revealed multiple life-threatening conditions. The deep laceration on the forehead, combined with unequal pupils and a low GCS score, pointed to a traumatic brain injury. This was a serious concern, as increased intracranial pressure could lead to brain herniation, a life-threatening condition where brain tissue is forced out of its normal position.

The femur fracture was another critical injury. The femur, or thigh bone, is the longest and strongest bone in the body, and a break can cause substantial internal bleeding, leading to hypovolemic shock. Applying a traction splint would help align the bone ends and reduce bleeding. The open fracture of the left arm also posed a risk of infection and further blood loss, requiring immediate stabilization and sterile dressing.

The distended abdomen indicated internal bleeding, possibly from damage to the liver, spleen, or other abdominal organs. This type of injury necessitated rapid transport to a surgical team capable of performing a laparotomy, an emergency procedure to identify and control the source of bleeding.

Throughout the transport, maintaining airway patency and adequate ventilation was paramount. The high-flow oxygen delivered via mask helped maximize oxygenation, but the shallow and rapid breathing suggested potential rib fractures or a pneumothorax (collapsed lung). Continuous monitoring with a portable pulse oximeter ensured we kept track of the patient's oxygen saturation levels.

Administering IV fluids was crucial in managing the patient's shock. Crystalloids, such as normal saline or lactated Ringer's solution, were used to expand the circulating blood volume and improve perfusion to vital organs. However, we had to be cautious about fluid overload, especially with the possibility of internal bleeding.

The pelvic binder served to stabilize any potential pelvic fractures, which could also be a significant source of blood loss. The binder helps to reduce the volume of the pelvic cavity, thereby decreasing hemorrhage and providing some pain relief.

The erratic heart rate and dropping blood pressure

indicated the patient was in critical condition, and we prepared for possible cardiac arrest by setting up the defibrillator. Medications such as epinephrine and amiodarone were ready for administration, following Advanced Cardiac Life Support (ACLS) protocols.

Upon arrival at the hospital, the rapid handover included all vital information: the mechanism of injury, initial findings, treatments administered, and changes in the patient's condition during transport. This information was crucial for the trauma team to continue the life-saving efforts without delay.

The paramedic's role in such emergencies extends beyond the immediate care provided. It involves critical thinking, rapid decision-making, and seamless teamwork to stabilize the patient and ensure they receive the best possible care en route to the hospital. Each call hones these skills, making us better prepared for the next crisis.

The job is demanding, both physically and emotionally, but the rewards are profound. Each life saved, each family spared the grief of loss, reaffirms our commitment to this challenging yet vital profession. The story of this patient, like many others, is a testament to the resilience of the human spirit and the unwavering dedication of those who answer the call in the darkest hours of the night.

CHAPTER FIVE

SHARK BITE

WHEN THE CALL CAME IN, the tone of the dispatcher's voice indicated urgency. It was mid-afternoon on a surprisingly calm summer day. The sun beat down relentlessly, casting shimmering heat waves off the asphalt as we sped towards the marina. The report was of a man bitten by a shark, currently in critical condition.

Arriving at the marina, I saw the chaos that had erupted on the pier. A group of beachgoers and boat staff crowded around a figure lying on the wooden planks. The patient was barely conscious, his pallor a stark contrast to the vibrant hues of the beach around him. The scene was a mixture of alarm and desperation, everyone uncertain of how to help.

The patient had a deep, jagged laceration on his left thigh, consistent with a shark bite. The wound was gaping and irregular, indicative of the powerful jaws and serrated teeth that had caused it. Blood was pooling around him, and I could see the telltale signs of hypovolemic shock setting in – his skin was clammy and cool, and his breathing was rapid and shallow.

First things first, I donned my gloves and did a quick primary survey. The patient had a weak carotid pulse, and his respiratory rate was elevated at about 30 breaths per minute. He was drifting in and out of consciousness, responding only to painful stimuli. I knew we had to work fast.

I grabbed the trauma shears from my kit and quickly cut away the patient's soaked and bloodied clothing to better assess the wound. The bite had shredded through muscle and sinew, exposing bone. The edges of the wound were ragged, and the blood was a dark, ominous red. I noted that the bleeding was both arterial and venous, with spurts indicating a severed artery.

We needed to control the bleeding immediately. I applied a tourniquet high on the patient's thigh, just above the wound. I tightened it until the arterial spurting stopped, though venous oozing continued. Next, I packed the wound with sterile gauze, applying direct pressure to stem the venous bleeding as much as possible.

In the ambulance, I secured an IV line, using a large-bore catheter to facilitate rapid fluid resuscitation. The patient needed fluids to combat the shock, so I started him on a bolus of normal saline. His vital signs were still critical, with a systolic blood pressure barely touching 80 mmHg.

As the saline flowed into the patient's veins, I did a secondary survey. There were no other obvious injuries, but the patient's condition was still tenuous. I monitored his vital signs continuously, noting any changes. His heart rate was tachycardic, hovering around 130 beats per minute, a clear indication that his body was struggling to compensate for the blood loss.

While en route to the hospital, I contacted the emergency department to give them a heads-up. I detailed the patient's condition, the suspected shark bite, the location and severity of the injury, and the treatment administered so far. I knew that getting the hospital team prepared would be crucial for the patient's survival.

I continued monitoring the patient closely, adjusting the flow of saline to maintain his blood pressure. I also kept an eye on his mental status. He remained mostly unresponsive, only moaning occasionally when the ambulance hit a bump. I noted that his skin was still pale and cool, classic signs of hypoperfusion.

The patient's respiratory effort began to weaken, and I knew we might need to assist his breathing. I prepared the bag-valve mask (BVM) and had it ready. I also prepared an endotracheal tube, just in case he went into respiratory arrest. Time was of the essence, and we had to be ready for anything.

The patient's condition remained critical but stable as we approached the hospital. I updated the emergency department with his latest vitals: heart rate still around 130, respiratory rate now assisted with the BVM, and a blood pressure of 90/60 with the continued fluid resuscitation.

We arrived at the hospital, and the trauma team was waiting for us. As we transferred the patient to their care, I gave a quick yet detailed handoff, outlining the injury, treatment, and current status. The doctors and nurses quickly took over, rushing the patient into the trauma bay for further evaluation and treatment.

The patient's prognosis was still uncertain. Shark bites, especially those resulting in severe blood loss and tissue damage, carried a high risk of complications. The immediate concerns were continued bleeding, infection, and potential damage to underlying structures such as nerves and blood vessels.

As the trauma team worked, I took a moment to catch my breath and reflect on the call. Despite the gravity of the situation, there was a certain rhythm and flow to the way we handled it. Training and experience had prepared us for moments like these, where every second counted and every decision could mean the difference between life and death.

Later, I learned that the patient had survived surgery. The surgeons had managed to repair the damaged blood vessels and clean the wound thoroughly to prevent infection. He remained in the ICU, but his condition had stabilized. It would be a long road to recovery, with potential for further surgeries and extensive rehabilitation, but he was alive.

Reflecting on the call, I realized the importance of teamwork and preparedness in emergency medical services. From the initial assessment and bleeding control to the fluid resuscitation and respiratory support, every step had been crucial. The coordination between the paramedics and the hospital staff had ensured that the patient received the best possible care in the shortest amount of time.

In the world of emergency medicine, not every story ends with a saved life, but this time, it did. The patient had a fighting chance, thanks to the quick response and skilled hands of everyone involved. It was a reminder of why we do what we do, and the impact we can have, even in the most dire of circumstances.

CHAPTER SIX

ACID BURNS

I HAD JUST FINISHED my third cup of coffee when the call came in. A 45-year-old male had sustained severe acid burns while working in his garage. As a paramedic, I've seen my fair share of gruesome injuries, but acid burns are particularly nasty. They eat through the skin, causing excruciating pain and potential long-term damage. I tossed my coffee cup into the trash and headed to the ambulance with my partner, Mike.

We arrived at the scene in under ten minutes. The patient's garage was a typical suburban setup—tools neatly arranged on pegboards, a half-finished project on the workbench, and unfortunately, a large, ominous puddle of liquid on the floor. The patient was lying on the concrete, writhing in pain, his clothes partially melted and his skin visibly red and blistering.

As I approached him, I quickly assessed the situation.

He was conscious but in severe distress. His breathing was rapid and shallow, and he was gripping his right arm, where the burns appeared to be the worst. I noted that his left leg and part of his torso were also affected.

First things first: safety. I needed to make sure that we weren't in danger of being exposed to the acid ourselves. I instructed Mike to secure the scene, ensuring there were no active spills or other hazardous materials around. We both donned our protective gloves and eye protection before getting to work.

I began with a rapid assessment. The patient's airway was clear, though his breathing was labored. Circulation was concerning; his pulse was rapid and thready, a sign of potential shock. His skin was pale and clammy, and the areas affected by the acid were already starting to swell and blister. I grabbed the saline solution from our kit and started flushing the burned areas, trying to dilute and wash away as much of the acid as possible. This step is crucial in minimizing the damage and preventing the acid from continuing to eat away at the tissue.

As I worked, I mentally ran through the list of potential complications. Chemical burns can lead to significant fluid loss and infection, not to mention the possibility of systemic toxicity if the acid was particularly potent. I needed to get him stabilized and transported to the hospital as quickly as possible.

After thoroughly flushing the burns, I applied sterile,

non-stick dressings to the affected areas. These would help protect the wounds from infection and further injury during transport. I also started an IV line to administer fluids, as the patient was showing signs of hypovolemic shock. The saline would help replace some of the lost fluids and maintain his blood pressure.

While I was working on the burns, Mike had taken a set of vitals: blood pressure, heart rate, respiratory rate, and oxygen saturation. They were all consistent with someone in shock, reinforcing the urgency of our situation. We loaded the patient onto a stretcher and secured him in the ambulance.

During the ride, I continued to monitor his condition closely. His blood pressure was dangerously low, and despite the IV fluids, it wasn't improving as much as I'd hoped. I administered a bolus of normal saline to try and boost his circulating volume. The patient's pain was also a major concern. I administered a dose of morphine to help manage it, being careful to titrate the dose to avoid any respiratory depression, which could complicate things further.

As we sped towards the hospital, I couldn't help but reflect on the importance of safety protocols when working with hazardous materials. This patient had likely been concentrating on his project, unaware of the danger until it was too late. It was a sobering reminder of how quickly things can go wrong and the critical role we play in those first few minutes.

The patient's condition remained critical but stable during the transport. I kept a close eye on his vitals and reassured him as best I could. I could see the pain and fear in his eyes, but there was also a resilience there—a determination to fight through the ordeal. It was a look I'd seen before in patients who had survived against the odds, and it gave me a glimmer of hope.

As we neared the hospital, I contacted the emergency department to give them a heads-up on our arrival. I provided a detailed report: middle-aged male, severe acid burns to approximately 30% of his body, primarily affecting the right arm, left leg, and torso. Vital signs indicated hypovolemic shock, IV fluids administered, pain managed with morphine. I emphasized the need for immediate decontamination and further stabilization.

When we arrived, the hospital team was ready and waiting. We transferred the patient to their care, providing a quick handover with all the pertinent details. They whisked him away to the trauma bay, and I could finally take a moment to breathe.

The adrenaline started to wear off, and I felt the familiar mix of exhaustion and relief that comes after a particularly intense call. I hoped the patient would make it through. The road to recovery would be long and painful, with potential complications like infection and scarring to contend with. But with the right care, there was a good chance he'd pull through.

As we prepped the ambulance for the next call, I couldn't help but think about the patient's family. I hoped they knew what had happened and were on their way to the hospital. They'd be in for a long night, filled with uncertainty and fear. I wished there was more we could do to ease that burden, but for now, all we could do was prepare for the next emergency and be ready to provide the same level of care and support.

Mike and I exchanged a few words about the call, but there wasn't much to say. We'd done our job, and now it was up to the hospital team. As I finished restocking our supplies, I thought about how each call is a reminder of the fragility of life and the importance of the work we do. It's a heavy responsibility, but it's also a privilege to be there for people in their darkest moments, offering a lifeline when they need it most.

With the ambulance ready to go, we climbed back in and waited for the next call. No matter what came next, I knew we were prepared to face it head-on, just as we had today. The life of a paramedic is unpredictable and often challenging, but it's also incredibly rewarding. Knowing that we made a difference, even if just for one person, is what keeps us going, call after call, day after day.

CHAPTER SEVEN

CRIMSON SNOW

I HAD SEEN my fair share of chaotic situations, but nothing quite like this. It was a crisp winter morning when the call came in. Dispatch had given us the rundown: a teenage boy had jumped off his roof into a snowbank, only to impale himself on a fence post. My partner and I exchanged looks—this wasn't going to be pretty.

As we sped through the snowy streets, I mentally prepared for what lay ahead. Upon arrival, we found the scene in front of a typical suburban house, a neatly shoveled driveway leading to a mound of snow where a group of frantic people stood. The patient lay still, skewered through the abdomen by a wooden fence post, the jagged end protruding obscenely from his back. The sight was enough to churn anyone's stomach, but we had a job to do.

The initial survey of the scene was critical. The patient was pale, his breathing shallow and rapid, a clear sign of shock. His parents were beside themselves, clutching at each other for support. My partner immediately started assessing his vital signs while I took a closer look at the impalement. The post had gone in through his lower left quadrant and emerged just below his right shoulder blade—a path that likely tore through his intestines and perhaps even grazed his liver.

With the snow beneath him rapidly turning crimson, we knew time was of the essence. The first priority was to stabilize the post to prevent any further internal damage during transport. Using a combination of gauze and rigid splints, we carefully immobilized the post. It was a makeshift solution, but it had to hold.

Next, we focused on the patient's vitals. His pulse was thready, and his blood pressure was dropping. We started an IV line to administer fluids, aiming to combat the shock. The heart monitor showed a tachycardia—a heart rate far higher than normal, which wasn't surprising given the trauma and blood loss. We administered a bolus of saline to help maintain his blood pressure, knowing full well that this was a temporary measure until he could receive definitive care at the hospital.

His breathing was labored, and we suspected a possible pneumothorax—a collapsed lung caused by the fence post puncturing his chest cavity. To counteract this, we prepared to insert a needle into his chest to relieve the pressure, a procedure known as needle decompression. With swift precision, we inserted the needle into his second intercostal space on the right side, immediately hearing a hiss of escaping air. His breathing stabilized somewhat, but he was still in critical condition.

Throughout this, I kept an eye on his neurological status. He was drifting in and out of consciousness, a concerning sign that he might be suffering from hypovolemic shock—a condition where severe blood loss leads to decreased oxygen delivery to the brain and other vital organs. We kept talking to him, trying to keep him awake and oriented, but his responses were minimal and weak.

Once stabilized as best as we could manage on the scene, we prepared for transport. Moving him was a delicate operation. Any jostling could exacerbate his injuries, so we used a backboard and lifted him carefully, maintaining the stabilization of the post and his spinal alignment. The snow and ice made the maneuver more treacherous, but we managed to get him into the ambulance without incident.

Inside the ambulance, I reassessed his condition. The patient's blood pressure had dropped further despite the fluids, so we added a second IV line to increase fluid administration. His skin was cold and clammy—a classic sign of shock. We covered him with a thermal blanket to prevent hypothermia, a common and dangerous complication in trauma patients, especially in such cold conditions.

I continued to monitor his cardiac rhythm. The tachycardia persisted, indicating ongoing blood loss. We had packed the wound as best as we could to slow the bleeding, but it was clear he needed surgical intervention. I could see the strain in my partner's eyes as he managed the airway, ensuring the patient was getting enough oxygen. We were both acutely aware of the ticking clock.

As we sped towards the hospital, the situation grew more dire. The patient's oxygen levels began to drop, indicating that despite our needle decompression, his lung injury was worsening. We decided to intubate—a procedure where a tube is inserted into the trachea to secure the airway and ensure adequate ventilation. It was a high-stakes procedure in a moving ambulance, but it was necessary.

I prepared the equipment while my partner positioned the patient's head. With practiced precision, I inserted the laryngoscope and visualized the vocal cords. The tube went in smoothly, and we secured it in place, connecting it to a bag-valve mask to manually ventilate him. His oxygen levels stabilized, but we knew it was a temporary fix.

Minutes felt like hours as we finally pulled into the

hospital's emergency bay. The trauma team was waiting, ready to take over. We briefed them quickly—penetrating abdominal trauma, possible liver injury, pneumothorax, hypovolemic shock. They nodded, understanding the gravity of the situation.

As the team whisked him away to the operating room, I felt a momentary pang of helplessness. We had done everything we could in the field, but now it was up to the surgeons. We cleaned up the ambulance in silence, each lost in our thoughts. The patient's survival hinged on the next few hours of surgery and intensive care.

Later, we learned that the surgeons had managed to repair the damage. The post had indeed torn through his intestines and nicked his liver. They had also found and treated a small arterial bleed in his chest. The pneumothorax was addressed with a chest tube, and he was now in the ICU, heavily sedated but stable.

The experience stayed with me long after the shift ended. It was a stark reminder of the fragility of life and the razor-thin line between survival and tragedy. The patient had a long road to recovery ahead, but he had survived. It was a testament to the teamwork and rapid response of everyone involved, from the dispatch operator to the surgical team.

Reflecting on the call, I couldn't help but find a touch of dark humor in the situation. The irony of jumping into what seemed like a soft, fluffy snowbank only to find a hidden danger was almost too absurd to believe. It was a story that would be told and retold in the break room, a mix of grim reality and the gallows humor that keeps us going in this line of work.

In the end, the patient lived, and while the road ahead would be tough, he had the resilience of youth on his side. It was a reminder of why we do what we do—facing the chaos head-on, making split-second decisions, and holding onto hope even when the odds are stacked against us. As I hung up my gear at the end of the shift, I felt a deep sense of gratitude for my partner, the medical staff, and the sheer will of the human spirit to survive.

CHAPTER EIGHT

SHALLOW LEAP

AS I NAVIGATED the busy streets of our city, my mind wandered back to the countless calls I had responded to over the years. Each one was different, each one a puzzle to solve, a life to save. Today's call came through the radio with an urgency that yanked me back into focus: a teenage boy had jumped from the Anderson Bridge into the river below. Anderson Bridge, a notorious spot where local teens dared each other to jump, was infamous for its height and the thrill it promised. However, recent droughts had left the riverbed shallower than usual, turning a daring leap into a dangerous gamble.

As our ambulance screeched to a halt near the bridge, I could already see the cluster of people on the riverbank, their faces a mix of horror and curiosity. We grabbed our gear and hurried down to the scene. The sight that greeted us was grim: the patient lay motionless, his legs twisted at unnatural angles, the water around him tinged with blood.

Initial surveys are always crucial. My training kicked in as I approached the patient. His breathing was rapid and shallow, a clear sign of shock. His skin was pale and clammy to the touch. I noted the absence of major head or spinal injuries, which was a small relief in this dire situation. However, his legs told a different story. The impact from the jump had shattered them both, with open fractures visible on his tibia and fibula, bones protruding through torn skin.

Time was of the essence. I signaled my partner to prepare the stretcher and spinal board. The first step was to stabilize the patient's cervical spine to prevent any potential spinal injuries from exacerbating. Once we had his neck secured with a cervical collar, we carefully rolled him onto the spinal board, taking extra care not to move his legs more than necessary.

The next critical step was managing the patient's airway, breathing, and circulation – the ABCs of trauma care. His airway was clear, but his breathing was labored. We administered oxygen via a non-rebreather mask, hoping to stabilize his oxygen levels. His pulse was weak and thready, indicating severe blood loss and shock. We applied pressure dressings to the open fractures to control the bleeding and then secured his legs with splints to immobilize the fractures.

As we worked, I couldn't help but notice the irony. The Anderson Bridge had always been a place of youthful exuberance and carefree leaps into the unknown. Today, it was a stark reminder of the consequences of those leaps. The low water level had turned what was once a thrilling jump into a life-threatening fall.

With the patient stabilized as much as possible at the scene, we loaded him onto the stretcher and moved swiftly to the ambulance. Inside, the cramped space became a flurry of activity. I established two large-bore IV lines to administer fluids and combat the hypovolemic shock. The saline solution flowed into his veins, a temporary measure to replace the blood he had lost.

As the ambulance roared to life, heading towards the nearest trauma center, I focused on monitoring the patient's vital signs. His blood pressure was dangerously low, a clear indication that his body was struggling to cope with the trauma. We began fluid resuscitation, increasing the IV drip rate in an attempt to stabilize his blood pressure.

While my partner drove, I contacted the hospital, providing a detailed report on the patient's condition and our estimated time of arrival. Communication with the hospital staff was crucial; they needed to be prepared for immediate surgical intervention upon our arrival.

Despite our best efforts, the patient's condition remained critical. His heart rate was erratic, a sign that his body was in severe distress. I administered pain relief medication, mindful of the balance between easing his suffering and avoiding further complications. Pain management was essential, not just for his comfort but also to help stabilize his physiological responses.

The journey to the hospital, though only minutes, felt like an eternity. I kept a close eye on the patient's oxygen saturation levels and monitored his cardiac rhythm for any signs of deterioration. The constant beep of the heart monitor was a lifeline, a reminder that despite the severity of his injuries, he was still fighting.

We arrived at the trauma center, and a team of doctors and nurses awaited us, ready to take over. As we transferred the patient to the hospital gurney, I gave a rapid but thorough handover, detailing his injuries, vital signs, and the treatments we had administered. The trauma team swiftly wheeled him into the operating room, where the real battle for his life would begin.

As I stepped back, the adrenaline began to wear off, and the weight of the situation hit me. The patient had a long road ahead of him, with surgeries, rehabilitation, and a significant risk of complications. Yet, he was in capable hands, and if anyone could pull him through, it was the skilled trauma surgeons and medical staff.

Reflecting on the call, I realized how crucial every second and every decision had been. From the initial assessment and stabilization at the scene to the rapid transport and continuous monitoring, each step was vital in giving the patient a fighting chance.

The Anderson Bridge would continue to be a spot of allure for thrill-seekers, but today's incident served as a stark reminder of the risks involved. As paramedics, we are often the first line of defense in the battle between life and death, our actions a critical link in the chain of survival.

The next day, I checked in on the patient's progress. The news was cautiously optimistic. He had survived the initial surgeries, and although he faced a long and arduous recovery, the doctors were hopeful. His youth and resilience would be his greatest allies in the months to come.

In our line of work, not every story has a happy ending, but this one, for now, was a win. And as I prepared for the next call, I carried with me the lessons learned and the unwavering commitment to be ready for whatever challenges lay ahead.

CHAPTER NINE

A SLIMY SITUATION

IT WAS one of those muggy summer evenings when the heat clings to your skin, and the air feels thick with moisture. My partner and I were stationed near the outskirts of town, hoping for a quiet shift. But as every paramedic knows, the unexpected is always just around the corner. The call came in just after 7 PM: a case of suspected poisoning. The details were sparse, but the urgency in the dispatcher's voice told us everything we needed to know. We were dealing with a serious situation.

The address led us to a quaint suburban home with a well-kept garden. As we pulled up, I noticed an elaborate picnic setup in the backyard, complete with a checkered blanket and what appeared to be a homemade feast. A man was lying on the ground, his face contorted in pain, while a woman nearby was doubled over, clutching her stomach. It was clear they were both in distress.

As we approached, I quickly assessed the situation. The man was pale, sweating profusely, and exhibiting signs of severe abdominal pain. His pulse was rapid and weak, and his breathing was shallow. The woman was in a similar state, though she seemed slightly more coherent. I grabbed my equipment and got to work.

First, I checked their vitals. The man's blood pressure was dangerously low, and his heart rate was through the roof. The woman's vitals were slightly better but still concerning. I asked them a series of questions to gather as much information as possible. The man, through gritted teeth, mentioned they had eaten snails from his garden. He thought they were edible and had wanted to impress his date with a unique culinary experience. Clearly, this was a decision he was now regretting.

Garden snails, unlike their culinary cousins, the escargots, can carry a variety of harmful bacteria and parasites. One of the most dangerous is the rat lungworm, Angiostrongylus cantonensis, which can cause a form of meningitis. Additionally, snails can harbor other pathogens like Salmonella and E. coli. Given their symptoms and the timing of their meal, it was likely they were suffering from acute food poisoning, potentially exacerbated by neurotoxins or parasites.

I relayed this information to my partner and we

began immediate treatment. We administered intravenous fluids to combat dehydration and electrolyte imbalance. Given their symptoms, we suspected they might also be suffering from neurotoxic effects, so we prepared to administer activated charcoal, which can help absorb certain toxins in the digestive tract.

The patient was beginning to show signs of neurological involvement: confusion, dizziness, and muscle weakness. These symptoms pointed towards possible neurotoxin ingestion. The woman was slightly more lucid but complained of severe abdominal cramping and nausea. We needed to get them to the hospital fast, but we also had to stabilize them as much as possible before transport.

I started an IV line on both patients, administering a bolus of normal saline to help stabilize their blood pressure and improve circulation. I also administered antiemetics to help control their nausea and vomiting. With the immediate measures in place, we loaded them onto stretchers and into the ambulance.

The ride to the hospital was tense. I monitored their vitals closely, ready to intervene if their condition worsened. The man's condition was particularly concerning; his pulse remained weak, and his breathing was shallow and labored. I placed him on oxygen to help support his respiratory function. The woman, while still in pain, seemed to be responding better to the fluids and medication.

En route, I kept a close eye on their neurological status, looking for any signs of deterioration. The patient's confusion was a bad sign. It could indicate that the toxins were affecting his central nervous system. I made a mental note to inform the ER doctors about the possibility of neurotoxin exposure, as this would guide their treatment once we arrived.

Upon arriving at the hospital, we quickly transferred them to the emergency department. I gave a detailed report to the attending physician, highlighting the ingestion of garden snails and the potential for neurotoxin or parasitic infection. The ER team took over, whisking them away for further evaluation and treatment.

Later, I learned that both patients had been admitted to the ICU. The man's condition was touch and go for a while. He developed symptoms consistent with meningitis, likely from rat lungworm infection, and required aggressive treatment with antibiotics, antiparasitic medications, and supportive care. The woman's condition, though serious, was less severe. She was treated for acute gastroenteritis and monitored for any signs of neurological complications.

Both patients eventually pulled through, thanks to the quick intervention and comprehensive care they received. The man faced a long recovery, dealing with the aftermath of the infection and the damage it had caused to his nervous system. The woman recovered more quickly, though she too had a harrowing experience that left her wary of ever eating anything from the garden again.

Reflecting on the incident, I couldn't help but find a bit of dark humor in the situation. The man's well-intentioned but misguided attempt at a romantic gesture had nearly cost them their lives. It was a stark reminder of the importance of understanding the risks associated with wild food consumption and the potential dangers lurking in seemingly harmless places.

As paramedics, we often find ourselves in the midst of life-and-death situations, navigating the fine line between humor and horror. This case was no different. It reinforced the unpredictable nature of our work and the critical importance of quick thinking, detailed assessment, and effective intervention. It also highlighted the resilience of the human body and spirit, capable of overcoming even the most unexpected and bizarre challenges.

As the shift ended, I made a mental note to research more about the types of toxins and pathogens that garden snails can carry. Knowledge is power, and in our line of work, staying informed can make all the difference in providing the best possible care.

CHAPTER TEN

PARTIED TOO HARD

THE NIGHT BEGAN like any other shift, with a mix of anticipation and routine as we prepared the ambulance for the evening's calls. The hum of the city was punctuated by the occasional wail of a siren in the distance, a reminder of the unpredictability of our work. Little did I know that this particular call would be one for the books, a case that would blend medical urgency with a touch of dark humor, highlighting the often strange reality of being a paramedic.

The call came in around 11 PM, a little earlier than the usual peak of Friday night chaos. The dispatcher's voice crackled over the radio, "Female, approximately 16 years old, suspected alcohol poisoning. Police on scene." My partner and I exchanged a glance. Alcohol poisoning in teenagers wasn't uncommon, but it always carried a certain gravity, a reminder of how delicate life can be at that age.

We arrived at the scene to find a house that had clearly been the epicenter of a raucous party. Strewn across the lawn were red plastic cups, remnants of snacks, and the unmistakable evidence of teenage revelry abruptly halted by law enforcement. A few disheveled teenagers were huddled on the curb, looking more annoyed than scared, while a couple of police officers were talking to a distraught adult who I assumed was the homeowner.

The patient was lying on the ground, partially propped up against a tree, her pale skin and labored breathing immediate red flags. As I knelt beside her, the smell of alcohol was unmistakable, and it was clear that she had consumed a significant amount. Her eyes were half-open, glazed over, and she was unresponsive to verbal stimuli. I quickly assessed her vital signs: pulse rapid and thready, breathing shallow, and a low blood pressure reading. Classic signs of severe alcohol poisoning.

Alcohol poisoning occurs when there is so much alcohol in the bloodstream that areas of the brain controlling basic life-support functions—such as breathing, heart rate, and temperature control—begin to shut down. It's not just about how much you drink, but how quickly you drink it, and this girl had clearly had too much, too fast.

I performed a quick Glasgow Coma Scale assessment, a standard tool for measuring a patient's level of consciousness. Her score was a dismal 6 out of 15, indicating a severe level of impairment. Time was of the essence. Alcohol poisoning can lead to seizures, permanent brain damage, or even death if not treated promptly.

We quickly moved her to the stretcher and secured her in the ambulance. My partner, a seasoned paramedic with a penchant for gallows humor, quipped about the hazards of teenage invincibility. It was his way of coping with the gravity of our work, a shield against the often harsh reality we faced.

As we sped towards the hospital, I began the necessary emergency care. The first step was to secure her airway. Alcohol poisoning often leads to vomiting, and an unconscious patient can easily aspirate, leading to potentially fatal respiratory complications. I positioned her in a lateral recumbent position to prevent aspiration and monitored her breathing closely.

Next, I started an IV line to administer fluids. Dehydration is a common consequence of excessive alcohol consumption, exacerbated by the diuretic effects of alcohol. Normal saline was the go-to choice to replenish her fluids and help stabilize her blood pressure. As the IV drip started, I could only hope that her body would respond positively.

Hypoglycemia is another risk in alcohol poisoning cases. Alcohol interferes with the liver's ability to release glucose into the bloodstream, and without sufficient glucose, the brain and other vital organs can suffer. I checked her blood glucose levels, which were indeed low, and administered a dextrose solution to address the imbalance.

Throughout the journey, I kept a close eye on her vital signs, noting any changes. Her pulse remained erratic, a worrying sign that her body was struggling to cope with the onslaught of alcohol. I applied a non-rebreather mask to ensure she was getting sufficient oxygen. Hypoxia, or low oxygen levels in the blood, can exacerbate the already dangerous situation.

As we neared the hospital, I prepared my report for the emergency department. A succinct yet comprehensive account of her condition and the steps we had taken would be crucial for the ER team to take over her care seamlessly.

Upon arrival, the ER team was ready and waiting. We transferred the patient to a gurney, and I gave a brief rundown of her condition. The doctors nodded, already moving to intubate her to secure her airway and prepare for gastric lavage to clear her stomach of any remaining alcohol.

As we left the hospital, there was a sense of relief mixed with the sobering reminder of how easily a night of fun could turn into a life-threatening situation. The patient's prognosis was uncertain, but we had done everything we could to give her the best chance of survival.

Later, I learned that the patient had been found unconscious by the police after they busted up the party. She had been left outside by her so-called friends, too scared of getting into trouble to seek help for her. It was a bitter pill to swallow, the reality of peer pressure and the fear of authority overshadowing basic human decency.

Alcohol poisoning in teenagers is a stark reminder of the need for better education and awareness. It's not just about telling kids not to drink but helping them under-stand the real risks and what to do if they find them-selves or their friends in trouble. The memory of that night, of a young girl teetering on the edge of life and death, is a poignant example of why our work as para-medics is so vital.

As for the patient, she survived. It took several days in the ICU, but she pulled through, thanks to the quick response and the tireless efforts of the medical team. When I heard the news, there was a sense of satisfaction mixed with a hope that she, and others like her, would learn from the experience and make better choices in the future.

Reflecting on that night, it's clear that every call is a unique blend of urgency, routine, and the unexpected. As paramedics, we navigate this complex landscape, bringing medical expertise and a touch of humor to bear in the most trying of circumstances. And sometimes, in those quiet moments between calls, we allow ourselves a moment of gratitude for the lives we've helped save and the lessons we've learned along the way.

CHAPTER ELEVEN

ALWAYS LOOK BOTH WAYS

WE WERE ROLLING down Main Street, the sun just beginning to dip below the horizon, casting long shadows across the bustling city. It had been a relatively quiet shift until the call came through: pedestrian struck by a vehicle, possible severe injuries. The dispatcher's voice crackled over the radio, and we immediately hit the lights and sirens, weaving through the traffic that parted reluctantly before us. As a paramedic, you learn to steel yourself for what you might encounter, but every scene is a fresh slate of unpredictability.

We arrived at the scene in under three minutes, but it felt longer. Cars had already started to back up, a sea of metal and rubber surrounding the point of impact. The crowd of bystanders had formed a loose circle around a figure lying prone in the street. My partner and I grabbed our gear and dashed over, my adrenaline already kicking into high gear.

The patient was a middle-aged man, sprawled awkwardly on the asphalt. He had been hit hard, evidenced by the significant dent on the front bumper of the sedan that sat, idling, a few feet away. The driver, a young woman, stood nearby, shock and horror etched on her face. But my focus was entirely on the patient.

My initial survey was quick but thorough, a practiced dance of assessment. He was unconscious but breathing, though shallowly. A large laceration on his forehead was bleeding profusely, the blood mixing with the dirt and grit of the street. His left leg was twisted at an unnatural angle, suggesting a likely fracture. There were visible contusions on his chest, possibly indicating internal injuries.

I signaled my partner to get the cervical collar and backboard. Given the mechanism of injury, spinal precautions were paramount. While waiting, I gently but firmly stabilized his head and neck with my hands. My partner returned, and we quickly and efficiently applied the cervical collar, ensuring his neck was immobilized.

Next, we did a rapid trauma assessment. I checked his airway first. His mouth was clear, no obstructions or fluids. Breathing was shallow and rapid, around 28 breaths per minute, and his skin was cool and clammy to the touch. His pulse was weak and thready, racing at about 120 beats per minute. The signs pointed towards hypovolemic shock, likely from internal and external bleeding.

We had to work fast. I applied a non-rebreather mask, setting the oxygen flow to 15 liters per minute to ensure he was getting as much oxygen as possible. Meanwhile, my partner cut away the patient's clothing to expose the chest and check for further injuries. There were significant bruises across the thorax, suggesting potential rib fractures and internal bleeding, possibly a pneumothorax or hemothorax.

With the cervical collar in place, we log-rolled the patient onto his side, carefully sliding the backboard underneath him before rolling him back and securing him with straps. As we moved him, I noted a distinct crunching sensation—crepitus—indicative of broken ribs. His abdomen was rigid and distended, raising my suspicion of internal bleeding.

We loaded the patient into the ambulance swiftly but carefully, continuing to monitor his vitals. Inside, my partner started two large-bore IV lines, one in each arm, to administer fluids and help counteract the shock. We hung normal saline bags and opened them wide, the fluid rushing into his veins to help maintain his blood pressure.

I hooked him up to the cardiac monitor, watching the EKG rhythm closely. He was in sinus tachycardia, his heart racing to compensate for the loss of blood volume. The pulse oximeter reading was low, around 88%, despite the high-flow oxygen. His blood pressure was dangerously low, 80/50, confirming the hypovolemic shock diagnosis.

To manage his pain and provide some sedation, I administered a calculated dose of morphine, careful not to overdo it given his compromised condition. We also applied a splint to his obviously broken leg, immobilizing it as best as we could in the field to prevent further injury and reduce pain.

Our transport time to the nearest Level I trauma center was about ten minutes. During the ride, I kept up a continuous assessment, watching for any signs of deterioration. His condition was precarious, a balancing act of maintaining his airway, breathing, and circulation—what we call the ABCs in emergency medicine.

I noted his pupils were equal but sluggish to react, a sign that his brain had taken a hit, likely a concussion or more severe traumatic brain injury. The bleeding from his head wound had slowed thanks to the pressure bandage my partner had applied, but it was still a concern. Every bump and turn of the ambulance had me hyper-aware of his fragile state.

My partner called in a report to the receiving hospital, detailing the patient's condition, injuries, and the treatment we had provided so far. This ensured that the trauma team would be ready to take over the moment we arrived, minimizing any delay in his care.

As we approached the hospital, his vitals remained unstable. His blood pressure hovered in the low 80s over 50s, heart rate still racing. I kept a close eye on the EKG, looking for any signs of arrhythmias. His oxygen saturation improved slightly with the high-flow O2, but it was still not where we wanted it to be.

We pulled into the ambulance bay, and the trauma team was waiting with a gurney. We transferred the patient swiftly, giving a concise handover to the lead trauma surgeon, detailing his injuries, vitals, and interventions. They rushed him into the trauma bay, and we were left standing in the bay, adrenaline still coursing through our veins.

I took a deep breath, the tension of the past fifteen minutes slowly releasing its grip on me. We began the process of restocking the ambulance and cleaning up, preparing for the next call. Each case is a testament to the thin line we tread between life and death, the critical minutes where our skills and decisions can make all the difference.

This call had been a brutal reminder of that reality. The patient had been critically injured, and despite our best efforts, his outcome would depend on the skill of the trauma team and the resilience of his body. As paramedics, we often hand off our patients not knowing their ultimate fate, but confident that we've done everything in our power to give them the best shot at survival.

The shift continued, as it always does, each call a new challenge, a new life in our hands. But the memory of the man hit by the car, his pale face and broken body, would stay with me for a while, a stark reminder of the fragility of life and the importance of every second in emergency medicine.

Back in the ambulance, I ran through the call in my mind, noting what went well and what could be improved. It's a habit I've developed over the years, a way to continually refine my practice and stay sharp. We checked our equipment, restocked supplies, and made sure everything was ready for the next emergency.

The city lights flickered as we rolled out, back into the flow of the night, ready for whatever came next.

CHAPTER TWELVE

THE SPA WAS ELECTRIC

THE CALL CAME in just as I was finishing my shift. It was one of those days where everything had gone relatively smoothly, and I was looking forward to clocking out. But, as every paramedic knows, the job doesn't end until you're truly off the clock. The dispatcher's voice crackled through the radio, and the details were sparse but enough to spike my adrenaline: a male, working in his spa, electrocuted after dropping a corded drill into the water. The address wasn't far, and we arrived in minutes.

Upon arrival, the scene was chaotic. The patient's wife was hysterical, but I blocked her out, focusing on the task at hand. The spa was an above-ground model, half-filled with water, and there, floating face-up, was the patient. My partner and I moved quickly, knowing that time was critical in an electrocution case.

The first step was to assess the scene for safety. The power source had been unplugged, confirmed by the patient's wife who was still shouting something I couldn't quite make out. We donned our gloves and approached the spa. The patient was unresponsive, and my immediate concern was the possibility of cardiac arrest, a common consequence of electrocution.

I checked for a pulse and found none. His skin was pale, and he wasn't breathing. My partner and I worked in unison, pulling him out of the water and onto a flat surface. I began chest compressions immediately, while my partner prepared the defibrillator. The patient's skin was clammy, and there were visible entry and exit wounds from the electrical current—small, charred marks on his hand and foot.

We attached the AED pads to his chest and stood back as the machine analyzed his heart rhythm. The mechanical voice advised a shock, and we delivered it. The patient's body jerked with the electric current, but there was no immediate response. We continued CPR for another two minutes before the AED advised another shock. We delivered it, and this time, we detected a weak but palpable pulse.

With a pulse restored, we moved quickly to secure the patient for transport. I inserted an IV to administer fluids and medications. An electrocution of this magnitude often causes significant internal damage, including potential cardiac arrhythmias, burns, and nervous system disruptions. The patient's vitals were precarious, with a rapid heart rate and low blood pressure. We needed to stabilize him en route to the hospital.

We loaded the patient into the ambulance, and I started monitoring his heart rhythm closely. He had a sinus tachycardia, which wasn't surprising given the trauma his body had just endured. I administered a bolus of saline to help with his blood pressure, and we placed him on high-flow oxygen to ensure adequate tissue perfusion. His breathing was shallow and irregular, so I prepared to intubate if necessary.

As we sped towards the hospital, I kept a close eye on his cardiac monitor. Electrical injuries often cause arrhythmias, and I was ready to intervene if his heart started to misfire. I noticed occasional PVCs (premature ventricular contractions), but nothing sustained that required immediate treatment. His blood pressure was inching upwards, a good sign that he was responding to the fluids.

Burns from electrocution can be deceptive; the external wounds might be small, but the internal damage can be extensive. I noted the areas where the current had entered and exited his body and estimated the potential path it took through his system. The entry wound was on his right hand, suggesting the current traveled through his chest, likely affecting his heart, and exited at his left foot.

Given the severity of his condition, I communicated with the receiving hospital, providing them with a detailed report of his status and our interventions. They prepared their trauma team for our arrival. In the meantime, I continued to monitor and manage his symptoms. His pulse was weak, and his skin was still pale and cool to the touch.

We arrived at the hospital, and the trauma team took over. I briefed them on the patient's condition, including the initial absence of a pulse, the defibrillation, and his current vitals. They whisked him away to the trauma bay, and I took a moment to catch my breath.

Back in the ambulance, I started the tedious but necessary task of restocking and cleaning. The adrenaline was wearing off, leaving me with a sense of exhaustion but also satisfaction. We had done everything we could in the field to give the patient a fighting chance.

As I was finishing up, I thought about the patient's situation. Electrocution injuries are rare but incredibly serious. The heart is especially vulnerable to electrical currents, which can cause immediate cardiac arrest or arrhythmias. The burns, though often small externally, can lead to severe internal damage, including muscle breakdown and organ dysfunction. Fluid resuscitation is crucial to manage shock and prevent kidney failure from muscle breakdown products.

Reflecting on the call, I was reminded of the importance of rapid intervention and the teamwork required to manage such emergencies. Every second counts, and having a well-coordinated response can make the difference between life and death.

As I headed back to the station, the radio crackled to life with another call. I sighed, knowing the shift wasn't over yet. But that's the nature of the job—never a dull moment, always another life to save.

Back at the station, I started to reflect on the specifics of the treatment. When dealing with electrical injuries, one of the primary concerns is the development of cardiac arrhythmias. The heart is incredibly sensitive to electrical disturbances, and even after initial stabilization, patients can develop late-onset arrhythmias. Continuous cardiac monitoring is crucial, both in the field and in the hospital.

Another significant concern is the potential for compartment syndrome. Electrical injuries can cause deep tissue damage, leading to swelling and increased pressure within muscle compartments. This can compromise circulation and lead to tissue death if not promptly addressed. The patient didn't show signs of compartment syndrome during our transport, but it was something the hospital would need to watch for.

Additionally, renal function is a critical aspect to monitor. The breakdown of muscle tissue, known as rhabdomyolysis, releases myoglobin into the bloodstream, which can cause acute kidney injury. Administering IV fluids helps to flush out the myoglobin and protect the kidneys, but further treatment might include medications or even dialysis if the damage is severe.

The burns themselves, while small externally, can cause significant pain and potential infection. The entry and exit wounds are the most obvious, but the path of the current can cause internal burns that aren't immediately visible. Pain management and wound care are essential components of the patient's treatment plan.

The patient's neurological status was another area of concern. Electrical injuries can affect the central nervous system, leading to seizures, confusion, or even long-term cognitive deficits. While the patient was unresponsive during our transport, it was unclear if this was solely due to the cardiac arrest or if there was additional neurological damage. A thorough neurological assessment and possibly imaging studies would be necessary to fully evaluate his condition.

As I finished restocking the ambulance, I thought about the importance of public education on electrical safety. Incidents like this are often preventable with proper precautions. Using ground-fault circuit inter-rupters (GFCIs), keeping electrical appliances away from water, and ensuring tools are properly maintained and used correctly can significantly reduce the risk of elec-trocution.

The next call came in, pulling me out of my thoughts and back into action. Another emergency awaited, another chance to make a difference. As we sped off to the next scene, I hoped the patient we'd just transported would pull through. In our line of work, we rarely get to know the outcomes of the people we help, but we always give our best, hoping it's enough.

The specifics of electrical injuries are fascinating and complex. The human body conducts electricity, and the severity of injuries depends on several factors, including the voltage, the duration of exposure, and the path the current takes through the body. Alternating current (AC), commonly used in households, is particularly dangerous because it can cause sustained muscle contractions, making it difficult for a person to let go of the source of the current.

When an electrical current passes through the body, it can cause both thermal and mechanical damage. The thermal effect results from the resistance of the body tissues, which generates heat. This heat can cause burns at the entry and exit points and along the path of the current. The mechanical effect refers to the direct injury to tissues as the current disrupts cell membranes and other structures.

One of the most immediate and severe consequences of electrocution is cardiac arrest, as we saw with this patient. The electrical current can cause the heart to go into ventricular fibrillation, a life-threatening arrhythmia where the heart quivers instead of pumping effectively. Defibrillation, which we performed on the patient, is crucial in these cases to restore a normal heart rhythm.

In addition to the heart, the nervous system is highly susceptible to electrical injuries. The current can cause direct damage to nerves, leading to symptoms ranging from numbness and tingling to paralysis. The extent of neurological damage can vary widely and might not be fully apparent until days or weeks after the injury.

Muscle damage, or rhabdomyolysis, is another serious concern. The breakdown of muscle tissue releases myoglobin and other intracellular components into the bloodstream, which can lead to kidney damage. Early and aggressive fluid resuscitation is key to preventing this complication, which is why we started the patient on IV fluids immediately.

The respiratory system can also be affected, both directly and indirectly. Direct injury to the respiratory muscles or the nerves controlling them can impair breathing. Indirectly, severe burns or trauma can lead to a systemic inflammatory response, causing acute respiratory distress syndrome (ARDS).

As we arrived at the hospital and transferred the patient to the trauma team, I knew they would be considering all these potential complications. They would likely perform a battery of tests, including blood work to assess his electrolytes and kidney function, imaging studies to evaluate internal injuries, and continuous cardiac monitoring to detect any arrhythmias.

In the ambulance, we often see patients at their most critical moments. Our interventions are designed to stabilize and buy time until they can receive definitive care at the hospital. This case was a stark reminder of the importance of our role in the chain of survival. Rapid assessment, effective CPR, defibrillation, fluid resuscitation, and careful monitoring—all these steps are crucial in giving patients like him a fighting chance.

Back at the station, I documented the call thoroughly, ensuring all details were recorded accurately. Each case adds to our collective knowledge and helps improve our response in future emergencies. The adrenaline had worn off, leaving me with a mix of exhaustion and a sense of purpose. We might not always know the outcomes, but every life we touch matters, and every call is a testament to the dedication and skill of paramedics everywhere.

Just as I was about to finish my paperwork, the

dispatcher's voice crackled through the radio again, signaling another emergency. I grabbed my gear and headed out, ready to face whatever came next. In this line of work, there's no rest for the weary, but the drive to help others keeps us going, call after call, day after day.

CHAPTER THIRTEEN

CHRISTMAS JEER

IT WAS a cold December afternoon when the call came through. Dispatch had received an urgent report: a man had fallen from a ladder while hanging Christmas lights. The caller, likely a frantic family member, mentioned he had landed hard on his shoulder and hit his head on the way down. The possibility of a traumatic brain injury (TBI) made this situation critical.

As we sped through the streets, I mentally reviewed the protocols for handling fall injuries. The risk of cervical spine injury, potential dislocation, and the alarming prospect of a TBI all flashed through my mind. The flashing lights and wailing sirens cut through the holiday cheer as we pulled up to the house.

The patient lay sprawled on the icy driveway, his face contorted in pain. He was cradling his right arm close to his body, a classic sign of a shoulder dislocation. His wife hovered nearby, eyes wide with fear but thankfully, keeping her distance to allow us room to work.

I quickly approached the patient, assessing the situation. His skin was pale, and there was a small, steady trickle of blood from a cut on his forehead where he must have hit the ground. His pupils were equal and reactive, a positive sign amidst the chaos.

"Okay, let's get to work," I thought. I started with a primary survey. Airway: clear. Breathing: rapid but unlabored, with a respiratory rate of around 24 breaths per minute. Circulation: his pulse was strong but fast, likely a combination of pain and adrenaline, clocking in at about 110 beats per minute. Disability: I checked his Glasgow Coma Scale (GCS) score, which was 14—he was alert and oriented but confused about what had happened.

With the primary survey complete, it was time to move on to more focused care. First, I immobilized his cervical spine with a collar to prevent any potential spinal injury from worsening. Falls like this often cause vertebral fractures, and the last thing we needed was to exacerbate a spinal cord injury.

Next, I turned my attention to his shoulder. The telltale bulge of a dislocated shoulder was obvious under his coat. Dislocations are intensely painful and can cause significant neurovascular damage if not addressed promptly. I palpated the area gently, confirming the displacement and checking for any obvious fractures. His distal pulse was intact, and he had good capillary refill in his fingers, suggesting that, for now, his circulation was uncompromised.

As I continued my assessment, my partner prepared an IV line to administer pain relief. With a dislocation and a potential head injury, controlling his pain was crucial, but we had to be cautious with medication due to the possibility of a TBI. We decided on a moderate dose of fentanyl, which would help manage his pain without overly depressing his respiratory drive or masking any neurological symptoms.

Once the pain relief was administered, we carefully maneuvered the patient onto a stretcher, ensuring his spine remained immobilized. His groans of pain were less frequent now, a sign the fentanyl was taking effect. The cut on his forehead, though not deep, required cleaning and bandaging to prevent infection, which my partner swiftly handled.

In the ambulance, I set up the cardiac monitor. His heart rate had dropped slightly to around 100 bpm, a good sign that the pain relief was working. His blood pressure was stable, and his oxygen saturation was at 98% on room air, so I decided supplemental oxygen wasn't immediately necessary.

Next, I performed a secondary survey, searching for any other injuries that might not have been immediately apparent. Aside from some minor abrasions on his hands and knees, there was nothing else significant. I continued to monitor his GCS, which remained stable, though he was still somewhat confused about the events leading up to his fall. I asked him basic questions to gauge his cognitive function, like his name, the date, and where he was. His answers, though slightly delayed, were accurate.

To manage his dislocated shoulder, we needed to keep it immobilized until it could be properly reduced at the hospital. I secured his arm in a sling and swathe, ensuring it was snug but not too tight, to avoid compromising circulation. Immobilizing the arm also helped alleviate some of his discomfort.

During the ride, I kept a close eye on his vitals and neurological status. I observed his pupils regularly, looking for any signs of unequal dilation that might indicate rising intracranial pressure—a serious concern with potential TBIs. Fortunately, his pupils remained equal and reactive throughout the journey.

The patient's wife rode with us in the front of the ambulance, visibly relieved but still anxious. In the back, the patient occasionally tried to move, grimacing with each jostle of the vehicle. I reassured him with a calm, steady presence, all the while keeping my senses alert for any changes.

As we neared the hospital, I prepared to give my report to the emergency department team. I detailed the mechanism of injury, our on-scene findings, the treatments we administered, and his current status. I made sure to highlight the potential TBI, the dislocated shoulder, and the stable but close-to-threshold vital signs.

Upon arrival at the emergency department, we transferred him to a hospital bed. I gave my report to the trauma team, who immediately began their own assessments. The patient's wife was directed to the waiting area, her face a mixture of hope and worry.

Once the patient was in the hands of the emergency team, we took a moment to clean up and restock the ambulance. These moments were brief, but necessary, allowing us to reset before the next call came in.

Throughout the entire call, we had managed to provide comprehensive and effective care, addressing both his immediate pain and the critical aspects of his injuries. The potential TBI was still a significant concern, but with his GCS stable and his vitals holding steady, we had done everything we could in the pre-hospital setting.

The dislocated shoulder, while painful and incapacitating, was straightforward in terms of management. Our priority had been immobilization and pain relief, both of which we had achieved. The true extent of his head injury would only be revealed with imaging and further assessment at the hospital, but our initial evaluation had shown no immediate life-threatening signs.

Reflecting on the call, I couldn't help but appreciate the mix of routine and unpredictability that defines emergency medical services. Each call is different, each patient unique, and every situation demands a blend of clinical knowledge, practical skills, and the ability to remain calm under pressure.

As we prepared to head back out, I thought about the patient and his family. The holiday season can be stressful, and accidents like these serve as stark reminders of the importance of safety in even the most festive activities. Our role is to be there when things go wrong, to provide care and reassurance, and to ensure that when someone's worst day arrives, they have the best possible chance of recovery.

This case, like so many others, reinforced the critical nature of our work. The combination of rapid assessment, effective treatment, and swift transport to definitive care is the cornerstone of what we do. And while the patient's journey was far from over, we had taken the first crucial steps in ensuring he received the care he needed.

As we drove away from the hospital, the radio crackled to life with another call. There was no time to linger on what had been; another patient needed us. And so, we headed out into the cold December afternoon once more, ready to face whatever came next.

CHAPTER FOURTEEN

NEVER PLAY WITH CLEAVERS

IT WAS a late Friday evening when the call came in. The dispatch reported a male patient in his forties who had severed three fingers while using a cleaver to cut meat. He had been drinking and showing off while making dinner when the accident occurred. We knew it was going to be one of those nights—gruesome, urgent, and messy.

Arriving at the scene, I immediately noted the chaos. Blood was everywhere—splattered across the kitchen counter, pooling on the floor, and smeared on the walls. The patient sat on the floor, his face pale and sweaty, clutching a makeshift bandage around his left hand. His right hand held a bloody cleaver, which he dropped as soon as he saw us. He had a wild, glassy look in his eyes, likely a combination of alcohol and shock.

I quickly assessed the situation. The first three fingers of his left hand were severed cleanly at the mid-phalangeal joints, hanging by thin strands of skin and tissue. Blood was still flowing freely despite his attempts to stem it with a dishrag. It was clear that we needed to act fast to control the bleeding and preserve the severed fingers.

First, I ensured that my partner, who was preparing the ambulance for a swift departure, had the trauma kit ready. I grabbed the sterile gauze and began applying direct pressure to the wound. The patient winced and groaned, but it was necessary. Hemorrhage control was our top priority.

I instructed the patient's friend, who had been standing uselessly in the corner, to find the severed fingers and place them in a plastic bag with some ice. This step was crucial for potential reattachment later on. He complied, albeit with a queasy expression, and returned with the fingers wrapped in a dishcloth.

With the pressure bandage in place, I elevated the patient's injured hand above heart level to reduce the blood flow. I checked his vitals: pulse was rapid and weak, indicating hypovolemia from blood loss, and his blood pressure was low. He was also tachypneic, breathing quickly and shallowly, a common response to shock and pain.

To manage his pain and anxiety, I administered a dose of fentanyl intravenously. Fentanyl, being a potent opioid analgesic, would help to alleviate the severe pain without causing significant cardiovascular depression. I also initiated an IV line with normal saline to replace some of the lost blood volume and prevent further shock.

Next, I needed to splint the injured hand to prevent further damage during transport. Using a SAM splint, I carefully immobilized his hand and fingers in a functional position, ensuring that the bandages were not too tight to impede circulation. The severed fingers, now in a plastic bag with ice, were placed in another bag to keep them clean and dry. I labeled the bag with the patient's details and time of injury.

Throughout the process, the patient was intermittently conscious, drifting in and out as the alcohol and analgesics took effect. I monitored his airway, breathing, and circulation constantly, ready to intervene if his condition deteriorated. The patient's friend hovered nervously, and I reassured him that we were doing everything possible.

Once we had the patient stabilized, we carefully transferred him to the stretcher and wheeled him out to the ambulance. The patient groaned again as we lifted him, but the fentanyl was starting to take the edge off his pain. I kept his hand elevated and ensured the IV was flowing properly.

Inside the ambulance, I hooked the patient up to the cardiac monitor to keep an eye on his heart rate and rhythm. I also checked his oxygen saturation, which was slightly low but manageable. I decided to administer supplemental oxygen via a nasal cannula at 4 liters per minute to support his breathing.

We began the transport to the nearest trauma center, a twenty-minute drive that felt like an eternity in these situations. The patient's condition remained relatively stable, though his blood pressure was still on the lower side. I instructed my partner to inform the hospital of our ETA and the nature of the injury, so they could prepare for immediate surgical intervention.

During the transport, I conducted a more thorough secondary survey to rule out any other injuries. Aside from some superficial cuts and bruises on his arms, likely from his frantic movements post-injury, there were no other major concerns. His abdomen was soft, and his chest was clear on auscultation. His pupils were equal and reactive, though his speech was slurred, likely from the alcohol and analgesics.

As we neared the hospital, I rechecked the patient's vital signs. His heart rate had stabilized, though still elevated, and his blood pressure was holding steady with the IV fluids. I ensured that the hand was still properly splinted and the bandages were secure but not overly tight. The patient's friend, who had ridden in the front with my partner, looked visibly relieved as we pulled up to the emergency department.

Upon arrival, we were met by the trauma team. I provided a detailed handover, outlining the mechanism of injury, the patient's initial condition, the interventions performed, and his current status. The trauma team swiftly moved the patient to a treatment bay, where the surgeons would assess the possibility of reattaching the severed fingers.

The patient was taken to the operating room for surgical debridement and an attempt at revascularization and reattachment of the fingers. The success of such procedures depends on various factors, including the time elapsed since the injury, the condition of the severed parts, and the patient's overall health. In this case, the quick action and proper handling of the severed fingers gave the patient the best possible chance.

As we cleaned up and prepared the ambulance for the next call, I reflected briefly on the evening's events. The patient had been fortunate in a sense—despite the severity of the injury and the complicating factor of alcohol, he had received timely and effective prehospital care. The surgical team would now take over, aiming to restore as much function as possible.

The job of a paramedic often involves managing

chaos and providing critical care under pressure. Tonight had been a stark reminder of that reality. We had done our part, and now it was up to the surgeons and the patient's resilience to determine the final outcome. With the adrenaline slowly wearing off, I prepared for whatever the night might throw at us next.

CHAPTER FIFTEEN
ACCIDENTAL SHOOTING

THE CALL CAME in as an accidental shooting, which was often code for a hunting trip gone awry. I was in the middle of my lunch break, but the adrenaline surged as I grabbed my gear and headed to the ambulance. Dispatch had mentioned it was a shotgun incident, so I braced myself for the worst. The drive to the scene felt like an eternity, though it was probably only a few minutes. We arrived at a clearing in the woods, where a small group of hunters was waving us down frantically.

The patient was lying on the ground, his face contorted in pain, clutching his right foot, or what was left of it. Blood was pooling around him, and I could see that a significant portion of his foot was missing. The scene was chaotic, with the other hunters trying to help but not really knowing what to do. I quickly took charge, assessing the situation and organizing the bystanders.

First things first, I needed to stop the bleeding. The patient was in obvious distress, sweating profusely, and his skin was pale—a sign of shock. I grabbed my tourniquet and applied it just above the knee. The bleeding slowed significantly, but I knew we needed to act fast to save as much of his limb as possible. I asked one of the bystanders to keep pressure on the tourniquet while I continued my assessment.

The wound was a mess of torn flesh, shattered bone, and shredded tendons. Shotgun blasts at close range do a lot of damage, and this was no exception. The foot was barely recognizable, with most of the damage concentrated around the midfoot and forefoot. I could see pieces of shoe embedded in the wound, along with dirt and debris from the ground. It was clear that infection was going to be a major concern.

I applied a sterile dressing to the wound, carefully packing it to control the bleeding further. I then secured it with a pressure bandage. My partner was already setting up the IV line, and I instructed him to start fluids to combat the shock. We hooked the patient up to a cardiac monitor, and his heart rate was through the roof —a combination of pain and blood loss. His blood pressure was dropping, another sign that we needed to move quickly.

With the immediate bleeding under control, I turned my attention to pain management. The patient was in agony, and I knew that controlling his pain was crucial not just for his comfort but also for stabilizing his vitals. I administered a dose of morphine, watching his face closely as the medication took effect. Gradually, his grimace softened, and his breathing slowed a bit.

We loaded the patient onto the stretcher, taking care to keep the injured foot elevated. Time was of the essence, but we couldn't afford to be reckless. Every bump and jolt could cause more damage or start the bleeding again. My partner and I lifted the stretcher into the ambulance, securing it tightly. I took a final look around the scene to ensure we hadn't left anything behind. The other hunters were still in shock, but one of them had called the patient's family to let them know what had happened.

Inside the ambulance, the atmosphere was tense but controlled. I gave the hospital a heads-up, providing them with a detailed report of the injury, our treatments, and the patient's vitals. They prepared the trauma team for our arrival. I double-checked the tourniquet and the bandages, making sure everything was still in place and holding.

The patient was more lucid now, thanks to the pain meds, but he was still in rough shape. I monitored his vitals continuously, watching for any signs of deterioration. His heart rate had come down a bit, and his blood pressure was stabilizing, but we were far from out of the woods. I kept the IV fluids going, ensuring he stayed hydrated and his blood volume was supported.

We hit a rough patch of road, and I saw the patient's face tense up again. I checked the bandages—still secure. I reassured him, more through actions than words, by making sure everything was running smoothly. I adjusted the oxygen mask over his face, providing him with a steady flow to keep his levels up.

In between monitoring vitals and adjusting equipment, I took mental notes for my report. The shotgun blast had caused an open fracture, with bone fragments visible in the wound. There was significant tissue damage, both from the impact and the subsequent contamination. The immediate concern was hemorrhage control, which we had managed, but the long-term issues would include infection risk and the extent of reconstructive surgery needed.

The patient started to drift in and out of consciousness, likely a combination of shock, blood loss, and the morphine. I kept talking to him, even though he wasn't fully responsive. Keeping a patient engaged, even minimally, helps in these situations. I monitored his Glasgow Coma Scale (GCS) score, which was fluctuating but still within a range that didn't overly concern me.

We were about fifteen minutes out from the hospital when the patient suddenly started to shiver—a sign that hypothermia could be setting in, exacerbated by the blood loss. I grabbed a thermal blanket and covered him, making sure to tuck it in around the injured leg without disturbing the bandages. I cranked up the heat in the ambulance, knowing that maintaining his body temperature was crucial.

The patient moaned softly, a reminder of the pain he was enduring despite the morphine. I considered giving him another dose but decided against it for now, mindful of the delicate balance between pain control and respiratory depression. I checked his oxygen saturation—still good.

My partner, who was driving, navigated the traffic expertly, using the siren sparingly but effectively. We communicated through quick glances and gestures, a well-practiced routine in high-stress situations. The road seemed endless, but the hospital finally came into view. I radioed ahead one last time, confirming our ETA and the patient's status.

As we pulled into the hospital bay, the trauma team was already waiting. We transferred the patient smoothly, briefing the doctors as we moved him from the ambulance stretcher to the hospital gurney. I detailed the initial assessment, the treatments administered, and the patient's response. The doctors nodded, taking in the information as they began their own assessment.

I stayed with the patient until they wheeled him into the trauma room. My job was almost done, but I still had paperwork to fill out and gear to clean. I took a moment to catch my breath, the adrenaline finally wearing off. The initial survey, emergency care, and transport were over, but I knew the patient had a long road ahead.

Reflecting on the incident, I realized how crucial every second and every action had been. From the moment we arrived at the scene to the transfer at the hospital, each step was a vital part of the chain of survival. The patient's life hung in the balance, and our quick thinking and decisive actions had given him the best possible chance.

CHAPTER SIXTEEN

TOXIC INJECTION

I REMEMBER the call coming in just as the sun was setting, painting the sky a fiery orange. The dispatcher's voice crackled over the radio, alerting us to a potential poisoning. It wasn't until we pulled up to the address that the severity of the situation became clear. The patient, a woman in her late twenties, had injected a toxic gel into her lips.

Upon entering the apartment, the scene was chaotic. The patient was seated on the living room couch, her face flushed and swollen, her lips grotesquely enlarged. Her breath was shallow and rapid, her skin clammy and pale despite the heat radiating from her body. The empty syringe lay discarded on the coffee table, a stark reminder of the gravity of her actions.

I immediately began my initial assessment. Her vital signs were alarming: a heart rate of 120 beats per minute, blood pressure of 160/90, and a respiratory rate of 28 breaths per minute. Her oxygen saturation was dipping below 90%, indicative of respiratory distress. I noted the swelling around her mouth, extending down her neck, potentially compromising her airway.

The first step was to secure her airway. I reached for the oxygen mask, adjusting it over her nose and mouth to deliver high-flow oxygen. Her breathing stabilized slightly, but the swelling was still a significant concern. We needed to act quickly to prevent it from worsening and causing a complete obstruction.

As my partner prepared the IV line, I gathered more information. The patient had injected the gel about an hour ago, hoping to enhance her lips. She hadn't anticipated the severe reaction. The gel, which she purchased online, was not FDA-approved and contained unknown substances, making it even more dangerous.

With the IV line in place, I administered a dose of epinephrine to counteract the swelling and an antihistamine to manage the allergic reaction. I also prepared a dose of corticosteroids to reduce inflammation. The patient's condition remained critical, but the medications would hopefully buy us some time.

We carefully transferred the patient to the stretcher, securing her in place before wheeling her out to the ambulance. As we navigated the narrow stairwell, I could see the concern etched on my partner's face. We both knew the importance of maintaining a calm demeanor, but the urgency of the situation was palpable.

Inside the ambulance, I connected the patient to the cardiac monitor to keep a close watch on her vital signs. Her heart rate was still elevated, and her blood pressure remained high, but the oxygen levels were improving slightly. I reassured her as I continued to monitor her condition, though her anxiety was evident.

During the transport, I began preparing for the possibility of intubation. The swelling was still a major threat, and if her airway became compromised, we would need to act swiftly. I readied the necessary equipment, ensuring everything was within reach.

As we sped through the city streets, I kept a close eye on the patient's response to the medications. The epinephrine seemed to be taking effect, as the swelling around her lips began to subside marginally. However, the risk of anaphylaxis loomed, and I remained vigilant for any signs of worsening.

The patient's skin was becoming mottled, a sign of poor perfusion, and her fingertips were cyanotic, indicating a lack of oxygen. I continued to provide high-flow oxygen, monitoring her closely for any changes. Her level of consciousness fluctuated, and I could see the fear in her eyes as she struggled to breathe.

I decided to administer another dose of epinephrine, hoping to further reduce the swelling. The corticosteroids were also beginning to take effect, but the patient's condition was still precarious. I placed a nasopharyngeal airway to help maintain her airway patency, a temporary measure that would hopefully keep her breathing until we reached the hospital.

Throughout the transport, I conducted a secondary survey to identify any other potential issues. Her pupils were equal and reactive to light, and there were no signs of trauma or other injuries. Her abdomen was soft, and there were no indications of internal bleeding. This reaffirmed that the primary concern was the severe allergic reaction and swelling.

As we neared the hospital, the patient's condition showed slight improvement. Her breathing had stabilized somewhat, and her oxygen saturation was holding steady at 94%. The swelling had not progressed, which was a good sign, but she remained at high risk for complications.

I radioed ahead to the emergency department, providing a detailed report of the patient's condition and the treatments administered. This ensured the receiving team would be prepared to continue her care without delay.

Upon arrival, we were met by a team of doctors and nurses who swiftly took over. As we transferred the patient to the hospital stretcher, I gave a concise handoff, summarizing her initial presentation, vital signs, interventions, and response to treatment.

The emergency team wasted no time, and I watched as they wheeled the patient into a trauma bay. I felt a sense of relief knowing she was in capable hands, but the gravity of the situation lingered. The patient's decision to use an unapproved substance had nearly cost her life, and the outcome was still uncertain.

We began the necessary paperwork and restocked our supplies, preparing for the next call. The adrenaline of the situation started to wear off, replaced by a somber reflection on the risks people take in the name of beauty.

As a paramedic, I've seen my fair share of emergencies, but this call was a stark reminder of the unpredictable nature of our job. Each day presents new challenges, and our role is to navigate them with skill, compassion, and a steady hand. The patient's fate was now in the hands of the hospital staff, and we had to trust they would continue the fight we started in the back of the ambulance.

In the end, the job is about making split-second decisions that can mean the difference between life and death. We are the first line of defense in medical emergencies, and every call is a testament to the dedication and resilience of those who choose this path. The patient's ordeal was a harsh lesson in the consequences of risky choices, and a reminder of the vital role we play in safeguarding lives, one call at a time.

CHAPTER SEVENTEEN
FRAT PARTY GONE WRONG

IT WAS JUST another Friday night, the kind that begins to blend together after you've worked as a paramedic for a few years. The calls we get on weekends are a predictable mix: bar fights, car accidents, the occasional heart attack. But that night, our dispatch received a call that set my adrenaline pumping—a college-aged man found unconscious, reportedly from alcohol poisoning after a hazing ritual. We were out the door and in the ambulance within minutes, the sirens blaring as we sped through the city streets.

Upon arrival, the scene was chaotic. The patient was lying on the floor of a fraternity house, surrounded by a mix of panicked and intoxicated peers. The unmistakable scent of alcohol and sweat hung heavy in the air. The patient was unresponsive, with vomit staining his shirt and the floor around him. His skin was pale, almost waxy, and clammy to the touch. My partner and I quickly assessed the situation. Airway, breathing, circulation—ABC, the cornerstone of emergency care.

His airway was partially obstructed by vomit, so I immediately grabbed a suction catheter and cleared his mouth and throat. His breathing was shallow and irregular, with a rate of about six breaths per minute—dangerously low. I could see his chest rising and falling, but it was clear that he was not getting enough oxygen. We applied a non-rebreather mask, delivering 100% oxygen, hoping to boost his oxygen levels while preparing to intubate if necessary.

Next, I checked his pulse. It was weak and thready, indicating poor perfusion. His heart rate was slow, around 40 beats per minute, and his blood pressure was alarmingly low at 80/50 mmHg. His body was struggling to maintain basic functions, a classic sign of severe alcohol poisoning.

I grabbed the glucometer and checked his blood sugar levels—sometimes alcohol poisoning can mask symptoms of hypoglycemia, but his glucose was within the normal range. We needed to establish an IV line quickly to administer fluids and medications. My partner skillfully inserted a large-bore IV into his arm, and we started a drip of normal saline to combat dehydration and help flush the alcohol from his system.

As the saline flowed into his veins, I ran through a

mental checklist of symptoms and potential complications. Severe alcohol poisoning can lead to hypothermia, hypoglycemia, and metabolic acidosis, among other issues. His skin felt cold, so we covered him with a blanket to help maintain his body temperature. I monitored his vital signs continuously, noting any changes that might indicate worsening conditions.

With the patient somewhat stabilized, it was time to transport him to the hospital. We carefully transferred him onto the stretcher and secured him in the ambulance. En route, I continued to monitor his vitals and prepare for potential complications. We started administering thiamine and dextrose intravenously—thiamine to prevent Wernicke's encephalopathy, a serious neurological condition caused by vitamin B1 deficiency, which can be exacerbated by heavy alcohol consumption, and dextrose to ensure his blood sugar levels remained stable.

The hum of the ambulance engine and the rhythmic beeping of the monitor created a backdrop for my thoughts. Alcohol poisoning cases can be tricky. Ethanol is a depressant, and in large quantities, it can suppress the central nervous system to the point where basic life functions start to shut down. The patient's breathing was still worryingly slow, and I mentally prepared for the possibility of needing to intubate if his respiratory status declined further.

As we sped through the city streets, I glanced at the patient's face—young, maybe in his early twenties. I couldn't help but think about the circumstances that led him here. Hazing rituals, often seen as a rite of passage in college fraternities, can sometimes spiral out of control, leading to dangerous and even life-threatening situations. But there was no time for reflections or judgments—my focus was entirely on getting him to the hospital alive.

Suddenly, the patient began to seize, his body convulsing violently on the stretcher. Alcohol withdrawal can cause seizures, but this seemed more like a direct result of the alcohol toxicity. I reached for the diazepam in our medication kit, quickly drawing up a dose to administer intravenously. The seizure subsided after the medication took effect, but it was a stark reminder of how fragile his condition was.

The hospital came into view just as his vitals began to stabilize somewhat. His breathing, though still shallow, had improved slightly with the oxygen therapy. His heart rate had picked up to a more regular rhythm, and his blood pressure was beginning to rise with the fluid resuscitation. We radioed ahead to the emergency department, providing a detailed report of his condition and our interventions.

Upon arrival, we were met by a team of nurses and doctors who took over his care. We transferred him to a hospital bed, and I gave a quick handover to the attending physician, outlining everything we had done so far. The doctor nodded, immediately ordering blood tests and preparing to administer additional treatments, including intravenous fluids, electrolyte correction, and close monitoring in the intensive care unit.

As we cleaned up the ambulance and prepared for the next call, I couldn't shake the image of the patient from my mind. His fate now rested in the hands of the hospital staff. The dangers of alcohol poisoning are very real, and it was a stark reminder of how quickly a night of fun can turn into a fight for survival.

Back in the ambulance, my partner and I reviewed the case, ensuring all our documentation was complete. Alcohol poisoning cases require meticulous record-keeping, especially when there are potential legal implications due to the circumstances of the hazing ritual. I made sure to note the patient's initial presentation, vital signs, interventions, and response to treatment in detail.

As we prepared to head back to the station, I took a moment to reflect on the medical facts that guided our treatment. Alcohol, once ingested, is absorbed primarily through the stomach and small intestine, entering the bloodstream and affecting the central nervous system. In cases of severe intoxication, the respiratory centers in the brain can be depressed, leading to respiratory arrest if not managed promptly. The liver metabolizes alcohol, but excessive amounts can overwhelm its capacity, leading to systemic toxicity.

The treatment protocols we followed were based on these principles. Clearing the airway and providing oxygen were critical first steps to ensure adequate oxygenation. The administration of intravenous fluids helped to correct dehydration and support cardiovascular function. Thiamine was essential to prevent neurological complications, and diazepam was used to manage seizures.

Our goal was to stabilize the patient long enough to get him to definitive care at the hospital, where more advanced interventions could be administered. Each step we took was guided by clinical guidelines and years of training, but in the back of my mind, I knew that every case is unique, and sometimes, despite our best efforts, the outcome is out of our control.

The call reminded me of the importance of public education on the dangers of excessive alcohol consumption, especially in environments like college campuses where peer pressure and the desire to fit in can lead to risky behaviors. While our job as paramedics is to provide emergency care, there's a broader role we play in advocating for preventive measures to avoid such scenarios in the first place.

As we drove back to the station, the city lights blurred into a mosaic of colors, and the adrenaline rush began to fade. I knew there would be other calls that night, other lives to save, and other stories to tell. But this one, the young man who was force-fed alcohol in a misguided ritual, would stay with me for a while—a stark reminder of the fragility of life and the critical role we play in those pivotal moments between life and death.

I took a deep breath, readying myself for whatever came next. The night was far from over, and as a paramedic, you learn to take each call as it comes, doing your best with the knowledge and resources you have. The patient was now in capable hands at the hospital, and I hoped he would make a full recovery. But for now, it was time to move on, to be ready for the next emergency, knowing that every call is a new opportunity to make a difference.

The familiar rhythm of the city's pulse was a constant backdrop as we rolled back to the station, ready to jump into action again at a moment's notice. Each call, each patient, each life hanging in the balance—it's what we signed up for, and it's what keeps us going, one emergency at a time.

CHAPTER EIGHTEEN
SOCIAL MEDIA CAN BE DANGEROUS

I WAS ON SHIFT, and it was an unremarkable evening, quiet for a weekend night. My partner and I had just finished a call and were restocking the ambulance when the dispatch crackled to life, reporting an incident involving a young woman who had sustained a head injury while attempting to film a video for Instagram. The details were sparse, but it was enough to get us moving.

When we arrived at the scene, the first thing I noticed was the car parked on the side of the road with its hazard lights flashing. The driver, visibly shaken, was standing by the passenger side door. Inside the car, slumped awkwardly in the front seat, was our patient. She was semi-conscious, with blood trickling down her forehead. It was immediately clear that she had struck her head with some force.

My partner and I quickly approached the vehicle, carrying our equipment bags. I did a rapid assessment as I approached, noting the patient's breathing and circulation. She was breathing on her own, albeit shallowly, and her pulse was rapid but present. My partner started to take a more detailed history from the driver while I focused on the patient.

The driver explained that the patient had leaned out of the car window to capture a video with her phone, not realizing how close they were to a roadside sign. They were traveling at a significant speed when she struck her head. The impact had caused an immediate laceration, and she had been dazed and unresponsive for a few moments before regaining some level of consciousness.

I assessed the wound on her forehead. It was a deep laceration, approximately four centimeters long, and bleeding steadily. Her hair was matted with blood, and I could see swelling already forming around the injury site. The nature of the impact and the visible swelling suggested a possible skull fracture, which was concerning given the mechanism of injury.

As I continued my assessment, I noted that the patient's pupils were unequal and sluggish to react, an indicator of potential intracranial pressure. Her Glasgow Coma Scale (GCS) score was 13, as she was opening her eyes in response to voice, was confused but able to respond verbally, and could follow commands to move her limbs. However, she was clearly in pain and disoriented.

I quickly applied a sterile dressing to the wound to control the bleeding. My partner and I decided it was essential to immobilize her cervical spine given the high likelihood of a significant head and potential spinal injury. We carefully placed a cervical collar on her to prevent any further movement that could exacerbate her condition.

Once we had her neck immobilized, we prepared to transfer her onto a stretcher. This process needed to be done with extreme caution. Any sudden movements could potentially worsen her condition if there were an undetected spinal injury. Using a scoop stretcher, we gently lifted her out of the vehicle and onto our stretcher, securing her firmly with straps to minimize any jostling during transport.

In the ambulance, I set up the cardiac monitor to keep an eye on her heart rate and rhythm, while my partner started an IV line to administer fluids and any necessary medications. Given her head injury, we were cautious about administering too much fluid, which could increase intracranial pressure. Instead, we aimed to maintain a careful balance to keep her hydrated and support her circulation without causing further complications.

I also placed her on high-flow oxygen via a non-rebreather mask. Although her oxygen saturation was within normal limits, the additional oxygen would help reduce any potential secondary brain injury due to hypoxia. Monitoring her vital signs closely, I observed her blood pressure, which was elevated – a potential sign of a Cushing's response indicating increased intracranial pressure.

During transport, I performed a more detailed secondary survey. Aside from the head injury, there were no other obvious signs of trauma. Her chest was clear with equal breath sounds, her abdomen was soft without tenderness, and there were no deformities in her extremities. Despite the apparent absence of other injuries, the head trauma remained our primary concern.

I monitored her neurological status throughout the journey. She drifted in and out of consciousness, occasionally mumbling incoherently. When she was awake, she seemed agitated and confused, likely due to the concussion and possible brain injury. We worked quickly but carefully, knowing that every moment counted when dealing with potential traumatic brain injuries.

As we sped towards the hospital, I contacted the emergency department to provide a report. I informed them of the patient's condition, the mechanism of injury, our initial findings, and the treatments we had administered. This allowed the hospital staff to prepare for our arrival and ensured that a trauma team would be ready to take over as soon as we got there.

The patient's condition remained stable during transport, though I was constantly vigilant for any signs of deterioration. Her vitals were monitored continuously, and I reassured her as best as I could, given her semi-conscious state. The trip to the hospital felt both long and short – long because of the urgency and short because of the critical tasks we had to perform.

Upon arrival at the hospital, we were met by a team of doctors and nurses who quickly took over. We transferred her to a hospital stretcher with the same care we had used to move her initially. The trauma team immediately began their assessment, starting with a rapid head-to-toe examination and ordering a CT scan to evaluate the extent of her head injury.

As we handed off the patient, I briefed the receiving team in more detail, summarizing her vitals, the treatment provided, and her responses during transport. The hospital team thanked us and quickly wheeled her away to the imaging department.

As we cleaned and restocked the ambulance, I reflected briefly on the situation. The incident was a stark reminder of how quickly a fun activity could turn into a serious emergency. The patient's decision to lean out of a moving vehicle, combined with the impact of the roadside sign, had resulted in a potentially life-threatening injury. It was a sobering thought, underscoring the importance of safety and the unpredictable nature of our work as paramedics.

Despite the gravity of the situation, there were moments of absurdity that couldn't be ignored. The sheer recklessness of the patient's actions – leaning out of a moving car to film a video – was a striking example of how social media could drive people to take unnecessary risks. It was a peculiar reflection on modern life, where the pursuit of online attention sometimes led to real-world consequences.

In the end, it was a successful call. We had managed to stabilize the patient and transport her safely to the hospital where she could receive the specialized care she needed. The initial emergency care we provided – from controlling the bleeding to immobilizing her cervical spine and monitoring her vitals – had played a crucial role in ensuring she reached the hospital in a stable condition.

We knew that her journey was far from over, and she would likely require extensive medical intervention and recovery time. However, our job was to manage the immediate crisis and get her to the hospital, which we had done effectively. The rest was now in the capable hands of the hospital team.

As we prepared for the next call, I couldn't help but think of the patient and hope that her recovery would be swift and complete. And perhaps, this experience might serve as a lesson – both for her and for others – about the importance of safety and the potential consequences of seemingly harmless actions.

The paramedic life was filled with such stories – a mix of tragedy, urgency, and sometimes a touch of the absurd. Each call was a new challenge, a new story, and a new opportunity to make a difference. And as we headed out for our next call, I was reminded once again of why we did what we did – to help, to heal, and to bring order to the chaos of emergency situations.

CHAPTER NINETEEN

HANDS UP...STUPID

IT WAS A SCORCHING SUMMER AFTERNOON, the kind that makes the road shimmer and the air feel like a heavy blanket. I was just about to take a sip of my lukewarm coffee when the call came in: a woman had cemented her hand to the road during a protest. It sounded absurd, and I almost laughed, but there was no room for amusement in this line of work. The dispatcher's voice crackled over the radio, and we knew it was time to move.

When we arrived at the scene, it was chaos. Protesters were scattered, some shouting slogans, others recording the spectacle with their phones. In the middle of it all, there she was—the patient—sitting on the hot asphalt with her hand embedded in a block of hardened cement. Sweat dripped down her face, mixing with dirt and tears. Her expression was a mix of defiance and pain.

We quickly assessed the situation. The patient's hand was entirely encased in cement, which had bonded to the road surface. This wasn't going to be a simple extraction. The first priority was to ensure her safety and manage her pain while we figured out how to free her. I knelt beside her, checking her vitals. Her pulse was rapid, likely a combination of pain and adrenaline. Her breathing was shallow, and she was on the verge of hyperventilating. I placed an oxygen mask over her face to help regulate her breathing.

My partner began setting up an IV line to administer fluids and pain relief. We chose fentanyl, a potent opioid analgesic, to manage her severe pain. The dose was calculated carefully—enough to alleviate her suffering but not so much as to cause respiratory depression. While the fentanyl took effect, we contacted the fire department to request a crew with a jackhammer. It was clear that conventional tools wouldn't suffice to free her hand.

As we waited for the jackhammer crew, we monitored the patient closely. Her hand was starting to show signs of severe trauma. The cement had dried and contracted, creating a vice-like grip on her fingers and wrist. The skin was pale and cool to the touch, indicating compromised blood flow. There was a risk of compartment syndrome, a condition where increased pressure within a confined space can cut off circulation and cause muscle and nerve damage.

I instructed my partner to elevate the patient's arm as much as possible to reduce swelling. We also wrapped a tourniquet above the elbow, not too tight, just enough to control the bleeding in case we had to deal with any lacerations once the cement was removed. In the meantime, we kept the patient hydrated with a steady flow of saline through the IV.

When the fire department arrived with the jackhammer, we coordinated the extraction carefully. The vibration and force of the jackhammer could cause further injury, so we had to be precise. The firemen worked diligently, chipping away at the cement while we shielded the patient's arm as best we could. It was a slow process, and the patient occasionally winced and groaned, despite the pain medication.

Finally, after what felt like an eternity, we managed to free her hand from the cement block. The sight was grim. Her hand was severely swollen, the skin mottled with dark bruises. The fingers were bent at unnatural angles, some likely fractured. There were deep abrasions where the cement had pressed against the skin, and her nails were cracked and discolored.

We immobilized her hand using a padded splint to minimize movement and further damage. The tourniquet was carefully released, and we monitored for any sudden changes in circulation. The patient was still in considerable pain, so we administered a second dose of fentanyl, ensuring she remained as comfortable as possible during transport.

As we loaded her into the ambulance, I reviewed the possible complications and treatments. The immediate concern was preventing infection, as the abrasions and open wounds were prime entry points for bacteria. In the sterile environment of the ambulance, we cleaned the wounds with saline and applied a broad-spectrum antibiotic ointment before wrapping her hand in sterile gauze.

On the way to the hospital, I documented her condition meticulously. The fractures would need to be confirmed with X-rays, but it was evident that she would require orthopedic intervention. Surgical debridement might be necessary to remove any necrotic tissue and ensure proper healing of the wounds. The disfigurement was likely permanent, given the extent of the damage, but the primary focus was on preserving function and preventing further complications.

Despite the seriousness of the situation, there were moments of dark humor that seasoned paramedics often share. It was a coping mechanism, a way to deal with the absurdity and tragedy we encountered daily. As I cleaned and dressed her wounds, I couldn't help but think of the bizarre nature of her predicament.

Cementing oneself to a road was an extreme form of protest, and the consequences were severe. For what, some silly protest? The thought lingered, but there was no room for judgment now.

As we neared the hospital, I prepared to hand over the patient to the emergency department team. I briefed them on her condition, the treatment administered, and the potential complications. They would take it from here, performing the necessary imaging and consulting with orthopedic and plastic surgeons.

Our job was almost done, but the image of her mangled hand stayed with me. It was a stark reminder of the fine line between activism and recklessness, and the price some people paid for their convictions. As the doors to the emergency room closed behind us, we cleaned up the ambulance, restocked our supplies, and prepared for the next call. There was no time to dwell on one case when another could come at any moment.

In the end, it was just another day on the job, another story to tell, and another reminder of the fragility of the human body and the unpredictability of the world we lived in.

CHAPTER TWENTY

SLING BLADE

AS I CLIMBED into the back of the ambulance, I mentally prepared for the call we had just received. The dispatcher had relayed that we were heading to the scene of a man who had sustained lacerations to his shins while mowing the grass. The tone of her voice had hinted at the severity of the situation, and I had a feeling this call would be anything but routine.

Arriving at the scene, I quickly assessed the environment. The mower lay on its side, a few feet from where the patient was sitting on the ground, clutching his legs in obvious pain. Blood soaked the grass around him, a vivid crimson contrasting starkly with the green. I grabbed my kit and approached him, noting the makeshift tourniquets he had tried to apply using strips of cloth. It was clear that the patient had tried to stop the bleeding himself but wasn't having much success.

Kneeling beside him, I first checked his airway, breathing, and circulation—our ABCs. His airway was clear, and he was breathing heavily but steadily. His pulse was rapid, likely a combination of pain and adrenaline. I moved on to assess his injuries more closely.

The lacerations on his shins were deep and gaping, with jagged edges that suggested the blade had torn through both skin and muscle. The bleeding was severe, but not yet life-threatening if we acted quickly. I noticed that part of the blade guard was missing, and a piece of metal lay nearby—likely the culprit in this unfortunate incident. It seemed the patient had removed safety features from the mower, possibly to make it more efficient, a decision he was surely regretting now.

I began by applying sterile gauze to the wounds to control the bleeding. The patient winced but didn't cry out, his face contorted in pain. As I worked, I could see the depth of the cuts more clearly. The right shin was worse off, with the blade having cut almost to the bone in one area. I carefully but firmly applied pressure, wrapping the gauze tightly and then securing it with bandages.

Next, I prepped an intravenous line to administer fluids and, eventually, pain medication. The patient's blood pressure was low, likely due to blood loss, and he needed fluids to maintain circulation. I selected a vein in his uninjured arm, cleaned the site, and inserted the IV catheter, taping it securely in place. I then hung a bag of saline solution and adjusted the flow rate to ensure he received a steady supply.

With the IV in place, I reached for a syringe of morphine. Pain management was critical not only for his comfort but to prevent shock. I administered a calculated dose, monitoring his response carefully. The tension in his face eased slightly as the medication took effect, but I knew we had a long way to go.

As we prepared to move him to the ambulance, I continued my assessment. His vitals were stabilizing somewhat with the fluids and pain relief, but the risk of infection from such deep and exposed wounds was significant. I covered the bandaged areas with an additional layer of sterile dressing to minimize contamination during transport.

We loaded the patient onto the stretcher, securing him with straps to prevent movement. My partner and I lifted him carefully into the ambulance, ensuring his injured legs were supported. Once inside, I connected the IV to the portable stand and positioned myself for the ride to the hospital.

During transport, I monitored his vitals continuously. His pulse and blood pressure were still concerning but had improved with the fluids. I documented everything meticulously—his initial presentation, the interventions we had performed, and his response to treatment. This information would be critical for the ER team once we arrived.

As we sped towards the hospital, I turned my attention to potential complications. The depth and severity of the lacerations meant there was a high risk of compartment syndrome, a condition where increased pressure within the muscle compartments can cut off blood flow and damage nerves and muscles. I palpated the area around the wounds, checking for signs of swelling or hardness. While his shins were understandably swollen, there was no immediate indication of compartment syndrome, but it was something the hospital staff would need to watch for closely.

I also considered the likelihood of foreign objects in the wounds. The jagged nature of the cuts suggested fragments of metal or debris could be embedded in the tissue. Cleaning and debriding these wounds would be a priority in the ER to prevent infection and further damage.

Throughout the ride, I kept a close eye on the patient's mental state. He was alert but understandably distressed. The morphine helped manage his pain, but I was cautious not to administer too much, balancing pain relief with the need to keep him conscious and responsive.

The patient's tetanus status was another consideration. Given the nature of the injury and the environment, there was a high risk of tetanus infection. I made a note to ensure the hospital staff checked his immunization history and administered a tetanus booster if needed.

As we neared the hospital, I prepared to give a handoff report to the receiving team. I reviewed the details in my mind, ready to provide a clear and concise summary of the patient's condition and the care we had administered. This handoff would be crucial to ensuring a seamless transition and continuity of care.

Upon arrival at the hospital, we were met by the trauma team. I quickly relayed the patient's vital signs, the nature and severity of his injuries, and the treatments we had provided during transport. The team moved swiftly, taking over care and guiding the patient into the trauma bay.

While the doctors and nurses began their assessment and treatment, I took a moment to clean up and prepare the ambulance for the next call. As I did, I reflected briefly on the importance of safety features and the consequences of neglecting them. The patient's injuries could have been prevented if the mower's protective guard had been in place.

The call had been challenging, but we had managed to stabilize the patient and get him to the hospital in a timely manner. Our swift response and the care we provided en route played a critical role in his initial stabilization. As I readied the ambulance, I felt a sense of satisfaction in knowing we had made a difference, even if the circumstances were less than ideal.

In retrospect, the case was a stark reminder of the unpredictable nature of our job. Each call presents unique challenges and requires us to think on our feet, adapting to the situation at hand. The patient's injuries were severe, but with the right care and timely intervention, he had a good chance of recovery.

As we headed back to the station, I couldn't help but think about the importance of preventive measures and safety protocols. Accidents like this one highlight the critical role they play in keeping us safe, whether on the job or at home. It was a lesson hard learned, but hopefully one that would not be soon forgotten.

The day wasn't over, and there were undoubtedly more calls to come. Each one would bring its own set of challenges, but we were ready, prepared to face whatever came our way. That's the life of a paramedic—unpredictable, demanding, but ultimately rewarding.

CHAPTER TWENTY-ONE
BAD OIL CHANGE

I STARTED my shift on an unusually sunny afternoon, eager for what the day would bring. I was barely into my second cup of coffee when the dispatch came through: a man had been crushed under his car while chasing an oil leak. The jack had failed. This was a Code 3, lights and sirens all the way.

Upon arrival at the scene, I could see the chaos. The car, an old sedan, sat precariously on a failed jack, its weight pressing down on the man's lower torso. A small pool of oil glistened on the pavement, a silent witness to the mishap. Bystanders stood around, their faces pale with horror.

We approached with caution, ensuring the scene was safe before diving in. The first thing we noticed was the patient's distress. He was conscious but clearly in excruciating pain. His skin was pale and clammy, a classic sign of shock. His breathing was rapid and shallow, indicating significant distress and potential internal injuries.

We quickly assessed the situation. The car had to be lifted off him before we could do anything else. With the help of the fire department, who arrived shortly after us, we managed to lift the car using a hydraulic lift, carefully stabilizing it to prevent any further injury.

Once the car was lifted, I did a quick primary survey. The patient's airway was clear, though his breaths were shallow and rapid, around 30 breaths per minute, suggesting respiratory distress. His radial pulse was weak and thready, an ominous sign pointing towards hypovolemic shock, likely due to internal bleeding. His abdomen was distended and firm to the touch, a tell-tale sign of internal hemorrhage.

We immediately placed him on a backboard with a cervical collar to prevent any spinal injuries from worsening. I administered high-flow oxygen through a non-rebreather mask to improve his oxygenation, while my partner established IV access. Given the severity of his condition, I opted for two large-bore IVs, one in each arm, to administer fluids rapidly.

We started a rapid infusion of normal saline to combat the shock. As we loaded him into the ambulance, I continued my secondary survey. His pelvis was unstable, indicating a possible pelvic fracture, a common and serious injury in such crush incidents. His legs were cold and mottled, with no palpable pulses in his feet, further indicating severe vascular compromise.

During transport, I closely monitored his vital signs. His blood pressure was dangerously low at 80/50 mmHg, and his heart rate was racing at 130 beats per minute, compensating for the low blood volume. His oxygen saturation was holding at 92%, not ideal but stable for now. I applied a pelvic binder to stabilize his pelvis and potentially reduce the bleeding.

As we sped towards the hospital, I prepared for possible complications. We had a chest decompression kit ready in case he developed a tension pneumothorax, a condition where air trapped in the chest cavity could collapse a lung and compress the heart, a life-threatening situation. We also had our intubation kit ready in case he lost consciousness and could no longer maintain his airway.

The patient's condition remained critical but stable en route. I maintained a close watch on his vital signs, reassessing his abdomen, pelvis, and legs for any changes. His abdomen remained distended, and he grimaced in pain with every bump on the road, but he was still responsive.

To keep him engaged and distracted from the pain, I asked him to squeeze my hand intermittently. He managed to do so, albeit weakly, which was a small but reassuring sign. His mental status was fluctuating, likely due to the blood loss and shock. I kept the fluids running at a high rate, hoping to keep his blood pressure from dropping further.

As we neared the hospital, I radioed ahead, giving a detailed report to the emergency department. I informed them of the mechanism of injury, our findings, and the treatments we had administered so far. They prepared their trauma team to meet us upon arrival.

We arrived at the hospital in record time. The trauma team was ready and waiting, and we swiftly transferred the patient to their care. I gave a final handoff report, emphasizing the severity of his injuries and the treatments given. The doctors nodded, understanding the urgency.

The trauma team immediately took over, rushing him into the trauma bay. I watched for a moment as they began their rapid assessment and interventions. His journey was far from over, but he was in the best hands now.

The patient had a long road to recovery ahead of him. The immediate concern was his internal bleeding and the potential for other hidden injuries. The trauma team would likely order a series of imaging studies, including a CT scan of his abdomen and pelvis, to assess the extent of the internal damage. Blood transfusions would be necessary to replace the blood he had lost.

In the back of the ambulance, I took a moment to

reflect on the call. It had been intense and demanding, requiring quick thinking and precise actions. Despite the gravity of the situation, I felt a sense of satisfaction knowing that we had done everything possible to stabilize him and get him to the hospital promptly.

The oil leak that had caused this entire ordeal seemed almost trivial in comparison to the life-threatening injuries the patient had sustained. It was a stark reminder of how quickly everyday situations could turn dangerous. As I cleaned up the ambulance and restocked our supplies, I couldn't help but feel grateful for the teamwork and professionalism that had made a difference today.

Calls like this one underscored the importance of being prepared for anything. Every day brought new challenges and opportunities to make a difference, and today had been a powerful example of that. As we headed back to the station, I felt a renewed sense of purpose and readiness for whatever might come next.

CHAPTER TWENTY-TWO

SOCIAL MEDIA CAN BE DANGEROUS 2

I ARRIVED at the scene of the accident with my partner, a bright and sunny morning suddenly turned chaotic. We parked the ambulance a few feet from the suburban house, sirens still wailing. The sight that greeted us was both familiar and peculiar: a group of teenagers, phones in hand, looking anxious and bewildered. One of them was furiously waving us over.

The patient was lying on the ground in the backyard, her face bloody and bruised. According to the onlookers, she had been performing a TikTok dance move when she slipped, lost her balance, and collided face-first with the concrete patio. As I approached her, I noted the severity of her injuries. Her face was a mess, with blood seeping from multiple lacerations, a possible nasal fracture, and severe swelling.

First things first, I needed to assess her level of

consciousness. She was alert and oriented, albeit in considerable pain. Her airway was clear, but I could see swelling and bruising around her nose and mouth. Breathing was labored, likely due to the pain and swelling, but her lung sounds were clear, indicating no immediate compromise to her respiratory system. Her circulation was stable, though her blood pressure was slightly elevated, which wasn't surprising given the trauma and shock.

I moved to stabilize her neck, in case of any spinal injuries. A cervical collar was applied quickly and efficiently. Next, I assessed her for other injuries. There were no apparent deformities or injuries to her limbs, and her abdomen was soft and non-tender. This was a classic example of focused trauma to a single area, in this case, her face.

The bleeding needed to be controlled immediately. I applied gauze pads to the lacerations, applying firm but gentle pressure to stop the blood flow. Her right cheek had a deep gash, likely requiring stitches. The nasal fracture was evident from the unnatural alignment and the copious amount of blood pouring from her nostrils. I pinched her nostrils together, trying to slow the bleeding while keeping her head slightly elevated to prevent blood from flowing back into her throat.

Once the immediate bleeding was managed, it was time to transport her. We carefully transferred her onto a backboard, ensuring her spine remained immobilized. She winced in pain, but there were no signs of neurological deficits. As we secured her to the stretcher, I noticed her pupils were equal and reactive, a good sign that there was no immediate intracranial pressure.

In the ambulance, I started an IV line to administer fluids and pain relief. A dose of fentanyl was given intravenously to help manage her pain without compromising her respiratory drive. Fentanyl is preferred in such scenarios due to its potency and relatively short half-life, allowing for better control of pain during transport.

The next step was to continue monitoring her vital signs and managing her symptoms. Her blood pressure was stable, though her heart rate was slightly elevated, likely from pain and anxiety. I kept a close eye on her oxygen saturation levels, ready to intervene with supplemental oxygen if needed. Fortunately, her SpO2 remained within normal limits, so no additional oxygen was required at that moment.

Facial injuries, especially those involving the nose and mouth, can complicate airway management. I had a bag-valve mask (BVM) ready, just in case her condition deteriorated, but for now, her airway was patent, and she was breathing adequately on her own. The nasal fracture posed a risk of airway obstruction, so I kept suction equipment on standby to clear any potential blood or vomit.

During the ride, I performed a secondary survey to ensure no injuries were missed. Her chest was symmetrical with clear breath sounds bilaterally. Her pelvis was stable, and there were no signs of other traumatic injuries. The primary concern remained her facial trauma.

Facial injuries are notoriously painful and can lead to long-term complications if not treated promptly. The patient's face had already started to swell, making her almost unrecognizable. I explained to her, in simple terms, that we were heading to the hospital where she would receive a thorough evaluation, likely including a CT scan to assess the extent of her injuries. I mentioned this not only to reassure her but also to ensure she remained as calm as possible, knowing that panic could exacerbate her pain and distress.

The ambulance ride was smooth, but the patient's condition required constant vigilance. Facial fractures can lead to hidden complications, including damage to the orbital bones, which could affect her vision, and the maxillary bones, which could impact her dental structure. I mentally ran through the potential injuries: zygomaticomaxillary complex fractures, Le Fort fractures, and isolated nasal fractures. Each had its own set of complications and required specific treatments.

Arriving at the hospital, we transferred her to the care of the emergency department staff. I provided a detailed handover, ensuring they were aware of her initial presentation, the treatment provided en route, and my observations. The attending physician nodded, understanding the urgency of getting imaging done to fully assess her injuries.

As the patient was wheeled away for further evaluation, I took a moment to reflect on the oddity of the situation. A TikTok dance gone wrong had resulted in severe facial trauma, a reminder of how quickly accidents can happen and the importance of being prepared for anything. Despite the unusual cause, the treatment followed the same principles we apply to any trauma case: stabilize, manage pain, and transport safely.

In the end, the day's call was a testament to the unpredictable nature of emergency medicine. From the initial scene assessment to the detailed care provided en route, every step was crucial in ensuring the patient received the best possible care. It was a reminder that, in this line of work, no two days are ever the same, and every call presents a new set of challenges to overcome.

The detailed diagnosis would likely come after a thorough evaluation at the hospital. Initial suspicion pointed towards multiple facial fractures, including a probable nasal fracture and lacerations requiring sutures. The treatment she received in the ambulance, including pain management, bleeding control, and stabilization, was crucial in preventing further complications. It was a stark reminder of the fragility of the human body and the importance of each step we take to protect and preserve life in those critical moments.

In the hospital, she would undergo a series of diagnostic tests, including a CT scan to determine the full extent of her injuries. Treatment would involve a multidisciplinary team, including emergency physicians, trauma surgeons, and possibly a maxillofacial specialist. The initial emergency care provided was just the beginning of a longer journey of recovery for the patient, but it was a crucial first step.

As I cleaned up the ambulance and prepared for the next call, I couldn't help but think about the strange circumstances that had brought us here. A simple dance, a momentary lapse in balance, had led to a serious injury. It was a reminder of the unpredictable nature of life and the importance of being ready for anything in the world of emergency medicine.

———

Continue with
Crazy Ambulance Stories: Volume 3

AFTERWORD

In the world of emergency medical services, we often find ourselves at the intersection of the extraordinary and the mundane. The cases described in this book, while narrated with a touch of humor, are rooted in real events where people experienced significant trauma and distress. It's essential to acknowledge the seriousness of these situations and the impact they have on the lives of those involved.

The humor interwoven throughout these stories is not meant to diminish the gravity of the incidents but to offer a glimpse into how paramedics and other first responders cope with the intense pressures of their work. Laughter can be a valuable coping mechanism, a way to process the unimaginable and maintain a semblance of normalcy amid chaos. However, it's crucial to remember that behind every anecdote lies a person who experienced pain, fear, and uncertainty.

In the case of the woman who slipped while performing a TikTok dance, the injuries sustained were severe and required immediate, skilled medical intervention. Facial trauma can lead to long-term complications, both physically and emotionally, affecting a person's life in profound ways. The quick actions of paramedics and the subsequent care provided by hospital staff play a critical role in the recovery process, but the road to healing can be long and challenging.

Emergency medical responders are trained to handle a wide array of situations with professionalism and compassion. Their work often goes unnoticed, yet it is vital to the health and safety of the community. The stories shared here aim to shed light on the realities of this profession, celebrating the resilience and dedication of those who work tirelessly to save lives.

It's important to approach these tales with empathy and respect for the individuals involved. The humorous elements serve as a reminder of the human aspect of emergency care—a blend of skill, experience, and a touch of levity to navigate the most trying circumstances. But let us not forget that every call answered is a person in need, and every injury treated is a life impacted.

To the readers, I hope these stories provide insight into the world of emergency medical services, fostering a deeper appreciation for the challenges faced by first responders. Remember the seriousness behind the humor and the real people whose lives were touched by these events. Thank you for taking this journey through the eyes of a paramedic, and may it inspire a greater understanding and respect for the crucial work they do every day.

ABOUT THE AUTHOR

Derek Chance is a highly skilled paramedic with over 15 years of experience in emergency medical services. Known for his quick thinking and calm demeanor under pressure, Derek has a proven track record of providing exceptional pre-hospital care in high-stress situations. He specializes in trauma and cardiac emergencies, and is dedicated to continuous learning and professional development. When he's not saving lives, Derek enjoys mentoring new paramedics and volunteering in community health programs. His commitment to patient care and his ability to stay composed in the face of adversity make him an invaluable asset to his team.

ALSO BY FREE REIGN PUBLISHING

WENDIGO CHRONICLES

MYSTERIES IN THE FOREST

STORIES FROM THE NICU

CRAZY MEDICAL STORIES

PAWSITIVE MOMENTS: LIFE IN A VETERINARY CLINIC

STORIES FROM THE NICU

VANISHED: STRANGE & MYSTERIOUS DISAPPEARANCES

DIAGNOSIS: RARE MEDICAL CASES

THE BIG BIGFOOT BOOK SERIES

THE MEGA MONSTER BOOK SERIES

LOST SOULS: 50 NATIONAL PARK DISAPPEARANCES

ON CALL: EMERGENCY ROOM STORIES

CURSED: TALES OF THE WORLD'S MOST HAUNTED
OBJECTS

CRAZY AMBULANCE STORIES

IN YOUR OWN WORDS GUIDED JOURNAL SERIES

www.ingramcontent.com/pod-product-compliance
Lightning Source LLC
Chambersburg PA
CBHW022040190326
41520CB00008B/667

*9 7 9 8 8 9 2 3 4 1 1 0 3 *